# Understanding Addiction

Understanding Health and Sickness Series
*Miriam Bloom, Ph.D.*
*General Editor*

# Understanding Addiction

**Elizabeth Connell Henderson, M.D.**

University Press of Mississippi
Jackson

www.upress.state.ms.us

Illustrations by Regan Causey Tuder.

Library of Congress Cataloging-in-Publication Data

Henderson, Elizabeth Connell.
    Understanding addiction / Elizabeth Connell Henderson.
        p.    cm.—(Understanding health and sickness series)
    Includes bibliographical references and index.
        ISBN 1-57806-239-X (cloth : alk. paper)—ISBN 1-57806-240-3 (pbk. : alk. paper)
        1. Compulsive behavior.   2. Substance abuse.    3. Dual diagnosis.
4. Addicts.   I. Title.   II. Series.
    RC533.H465  2000
    362.29—dc21                                        00-042856

British Library Cataloging-in-Publication Data available

# Contents

# Introduction

Who has woe? Who has sorrow? Who has strife? Who has
complaints? Who has needless bruises? Who has bloodshot eyes?

Those who linger over wine, who go to sample bowls of
mixed wine.

Do not gaze at wine when it is red, when it sparkles in the
cup, when it goes down smoothly!

In the end it bites like a snake and poisons like a viper.

Your eyes will see strange sights and your mind imagine con-
fusing things.

You will be like one sleeping of the high seas, lying on top of
the rigging.

"They hit me," you will say, "but I'm not hurt! They beat me,
but I don't feel it! When will I wake up so I can find another
drink?"

—Proverbs 23:29–35, New International Version

Addiction is nothing new, as we can see from the above
quotation, in which the biblical writer paints a hauntingly
accurate picture of the devastation caused by alcohol addiction. Alcoholism, drug addiction, and addictive behaviors
affect every group at every level in our society. In the United
States, one out of four people has a parent, child, or sibling
who is addicted. In 1995 the National Institutes of Health
estimated the economic cost of alcohol and drug abuse at
over $240 billion. Lost productivity, illness, premature death,
and health care expenditures are all part of this picture, as
are costs associated with motor vehicle accidents and with
crime and incarceration. The emotional and social damage

is immeasurable. Abuse of alcohol and drugs disrupts personal development, relationships, and families, corrupting the very fabric of society. Addiction to nicotine is a problem of massive proportions, and the difficulty of shaking that habit is familiar to millions. Behavioral addictions include pathological gambling and sex and compulsive overeating. Most of us are affected, directly or indirectly, by addiction or its consequences on others.

We are familiar with the image of the skid row wino and the strung-out junkie, but addicts don't usually look or behave like that; they are more likely to resemble your next-door neighbor. They are often accomplished people, and many have achieved fame. In recent years, public figures have become more open about their problems with addiction. Betty Ford, the wife of former president Gerald Ford, struggled with alcoholism, then dedicated her life to establishing an addiction treatment center. Golfer John Daly also talked of his problems with alcoholism, as did the baseball hall of famer Mickey Mantle before his death from the physical consequences of addiction.

Our knowledge of the biology of addiction has grown tremendously in recent years. We have learned that the addicted brain does not function normally and that it is impossible to separate the brain's biological function from a person's psychology and will. Clinicians who treat addiction know that there is no one perspective or approach that is correct. Recovery for addicted people and their families involves physical healing, behavioral changes, relational reconciliation, and psychological and spiritual growth. This book brings those various aspects together to provide the reader with a useful working understanding of the problem of addiction and a basis for continued learning.

As a practicing psychiatrist and addiction specialist, I believe that arming the patient and family with information about an illness is essential for success in treatment. It is wise to know your enemy. In this book, I will attempt to provide a comprehensive overview of the problem of addiction from several perspectives, including that of the addict, the addict's family, and the treating clinician. As you learn about addiction, you will find that there are no simple answers and no routine cases.

I begin by answering the question "What is addiction?" When does casual use become something more? How much is too much? Why are some people able to drink socially and maintain control, while others become alcoholics? Why can't the alcoholic or addict just straighten up and exert some will power? How is it that some people can just put it down while others continue to the point of destruction or death?

After discussing who gets addicted and why, I explain the biological basis of addiction and just what it is that makes a substance addictive. I look at a typical course of addiction and explore the pathway to recovery. Since addiction affects the whole family, I describe how family members can help. I explore the topic of recovery, discussing some of the techniques and strategies that are used to help addicts. Sometimes a psychiatric disorder or severe mental illness coexists with addiction, and I look at the problems that accompany such a dual diagnosis. Pathological gambling, sexual addiction, and other compulsive behaviors that are behavioral addictions are also discussed. Because addiction is a major personal, family, and social problem, it is being studied in many laboratories, and I end the book by reporting on promising new research. The appendices give some history on the regulation of addictive substances and provide sources for further information.

When people discuss addiction, they often assume that there is a difference between alcoholism and addiction to other drugs. Although some important differences between alcohol addiction and drug addiction do exist, there are many similarities. When I examine the basic nature of addiction, alcohol and drugs are considered interchangeable, and the term "addict" is used to denote both the alcoholic and the drug addict, because the basic biological and psychological processes of addictive disease are the same for both.

As a result of the social changes that occurred during the 1960s and 1970s, it is more common than it was in earlier times for people to have used multiple drugs in addition to alcohol. The social and demographic differences between alcoholics and drug addicts have also diminished. But the basic nature of addiction is the same across categories of substances and shares common characteristics with compulsive behavior disorders such as pathological gambling. I will point out any important differences among substances; otherwise the reader may assume that the point being made regarding one could apply to any other.

*Understanding Addiction* gives an overview of an immensely complex subject in a form that is accessible to readers with no medical background. Addicts and their families will find it a useful resource in their efforts at recovery. Anyone who works with people will encounter addiction. Personnel directors, law enforcement and correctional officers, lawyers, social workers, teachers, pastors, managers, and legislators frequently face the problem of addiction and its effects and should find this book a helpful reference. The Web sites listed in appendix B make available much more detailed information for those interested in further study.

It is my hope that *Understanding Addiction* will help in the struggle to prevent and treat this pervasive and perplexing disorder.

# Understanding Addiction

# I. What Is Addiction?

How do you know if you have a problem with addiction?
How do you know if a loved one does? How much is too
much? At what point does social drinking become problem
drinking, and when does problem drinking become alcoholism? What about illegal substances? Are you an addict
if you use them simply because they're illegal? I am going to
try to provide a useful way to answer these questions, and I'll
also look at why it has been such a problem to come up with
a definition of addiction.

A joke that was being told around addiction treatment
facilities a while ago went like this: If you want to find out
whether somebody is alcoholic, follow him into a bar at
happy hour. When he's not looking, drop a dead fly on top
of his beer. If he's a social drinker, he'll leave it alone and go
on talking. If he's a problem drinker, he'll wait till no one is
looking, then flick the fly off. But if he's alcoholic, he'll wring
that sucker out . . .

Since this method of diagnosis is probably not practical in
the general clinical setting, clinicians have developed several
questionnaires that are used to determine whether someone is
addicted. The shortest, and one of the most accurate, is the
CAGE questionnaire, which applies to alcohol.

The CAGE questionnaire consists of four questions featuring key words that start with the letters C, A, G, and E.
A positive answer to at least one question suggests a problem
with alcohol. The CAGE questionnaire is not standardized
for use with other substances or with addictive behaviors, but
a positive answer to C, A, or G regarding drugs is a strong
indication that there is a problem.

The CAGE Questionnaire

C: Have you ever felt you ought to *c*ut down on your drinking [drug use]?

A: Have people ever *a*nnoyed you by criticizing your drinking [drug use]?

G: Have you ever felt bad or *g*uilty about your drinking [drug use]?

E: Have you ever had a drink (*e*ye-opener) first thing in the morning to steady your nerves or get rid of a hangover?

Although several other screening questionnaires have been developed, including the Michigan Alcohol Screening Test (MAST), the Substance Abuse Subtle Screening Inventory (SASSI), and the Addiction Severity Index (ASI), the simple common sense approach of asking people if they have ever had any problems associated with their drinking or drug use probably identifies better than 90 percent of those with addiction.

Denial is a psychological defense mechanism that is found almost universally in people with addiction. We will look more closely at this phenomenon in chapter 5, but I mention it here because denial is responsible for a lot of the confusion that abounds in trying to answer the question "Am I an addict?" or "Is my (spouse, child, parent) an addict?" Denial is a person's ability to ignore negative consequences in order to be able to continue to use the substance in question. It is ironic that this characteristic sign of addiction is probably what causes the most problems with diagnosis in the day-to-day clinical setting.

People who are truly addicted can come up with an endless variety of reasons and justifications for the bad consequences of the addiction and also with reasons why the label "addicted" doesn't apply in their case. So if you are worrying about a family member and show him or her the CAGE questionnaire, don't expect to get honest answers. But if you wondering if you yourself have a problem with addiction, you probably know the answer deep down. Denial is usually not complete. Most people with addictions are well aware of the feeling of being caught between a rock and a hard place, knowing that the addiction is causing problems but not knowing how to live life without it.

If you've answered "yes" to the questions in the CAGE questionnaire, and you think you're an addict, go ahead and turn to chapter 7 and read about recovery. Before you go any further in your study of this problem, you need to know that there is a way out and how to find it.

### Defining the Disease of Addiction

Identifying the exact point at which the use of a substance constitutes an addiction ought to be easy, but it is not. Confusion arises because we are limited to observing and describing behaviors, when what we are really trying to define involves a change in the way the brain functions as a result of exposure to an addicting substance. It's the same problem that appears in the story of the three blind men and the elephant. One man feels the elephant's ears and concludes that the creature is broad, thin, and waving like a leaf in the wind. Another feels the elephant's trunk and believes that he is touching something long and sinuous, like a snake. The third feels the elephant's leg, and notes that it is chunky and sturdy, resembling the trunk of a tree. All three are correct, but none has discovered the true nature of the elephant. Addiction is a complicated condition, with biological, physiological, psychological, behavioral, and spiritual aspects. For this reason it is best to think of alcoholism and drug addiction as multifaceted disorders, only one of which is the compulsive use of the addicting substance.

In 1972 the National Council on Alcoholism and Drug Dependence convened a group of researchers and clinicians to propose a broad working definition of alcoholism. They came up with the following: "Alcoholism is a primary, chronic disease with genetic, psychosocial, and environmental factors influencing its development and manifestations. The disease is often progressive and fatal. It is characterized by impaired control over drinking, preoccupation with the drug alcohol, use of alcohol despite adverse consequences, and distortions in thinking, most notably denial. Each of these symptoms may be continuous or periodic" (*Journal of the American Medical Association* 268, no. 8 [1972]: 1012–13). This statement encompasses several aspects of the disorder of alcoholism, and applies also to drug addiction. The two key elements that will constitute our working definition of addiction are (1) *loss of control* over the use of the substance, and (2) continued use *despite negative consequences.*

Defining addiction in the abstract is hard enough. Diagnosing addiction can be even more difficult. In extreme cases the diagnosis of addiction is obvious—the street addict who commits crimes in order to support the addiction, or the skid-row alcoholic. But what about the business executive who has two or three drinks—never more—every evening on the train home from work, but has withdrawal symptoms after elective surgery when his routine is disrupted? Or the church deacon who mostly shuns alcohol but several times a year goes on out-of-town benders for a week or so? Or the person who has one arrest for driving under the influence (DUI) and is sent by the court for alcohol and drug assessment?

The mere use of substances—even to excess—is not enough to diagnose addiction, so we look for behavioral clues. The *Diagnostic and Statistical Manual,* 4th edition (*DSM-IV*) is the current standard for diagnosis that is used by most mental health professionals, and it contains a working definition of addiction (fig.1.1). Interestingly, the manual does not use the term "addiction"; instead, the terms "abuse" and "dependence" are defined. Either abuse or dependence is present when the use of the substance continues despite negative consequences, interferes with important obligations,

FIG. I.I. *Diagnostic and Statistical Manual*, 4th edition

*Criteria for Substance Abuse*

A. A maladaptive pattern of substance use leading to clinically significant impairment or distress, as manifested by one (or more) of the following, occurring within a 12-month period:

1) recurrent substance use resulting in a failure to fulfill major role obligations at work, school, or home (e.g., repeated absences or poor work performance related to substance use; substance-related absences, suspensions, or expulsions from school; neglect of children or household)

2) recurrent substance use in situations in which it is physically hazardous (e.g., driving an automobile or operating a machine when impaired by substance use)

3) recurrent substance-related legal problems (e.g., arrests for substance-related disorderly conduct)

4) continued substance use despite having persistent or recurrent social or interpersonal problems caused or exacerbated by the effects of the substance (e.g., arguments with spouse about consequences of intoxication, physical fights)

B. The symptoms have never met the criteria for substance dependence for this class of substance.

*Criteria for Substance Dependence*

A maladaptive pattern of substance use, leading to clinically significant impairment or distress, as manifested by three (or more) of the following, occurring at any time in the same 12-month period:

1) tolerance, as defined by either of the following: (a) a need for markedly increased amounts of the substance to achieve intoxication or desired effect, (b) markedly diminished effect with continued use of the same amount of the substance

2) withdrawal, as manifested by either of the following: (a) the characteristic withdrawal syndrome for the substance, (b) the same (or a closely related) substance is taken to relieve or avoid withdrawal symptoms

*continued*

FIG. I.I.  *Continued*

3) the substance is often taken in larger amounts or over a longer period than was intended

4) there is persistent desire or unsuccessful efforts to cut down or control substance use

5) a great deal of time is spent in activities necessary to obtain the substance (e.g., visiting multiple doctors or driving long distances), use the substance (e.g., chain smoking), or recover from its effects

6) important social, occupational, or recreational activities are given up or reduced because of substance use

7) the substance use is continued despite knowledge of having a persistent or recurrent physical or psychological problem that is likely to have been caused or exacerbated by the substance (e.g., current cocaine use despite recognition of cocaine-induced depression, or continued drinking despite recognition that an ulcer was made worse by alcohol consumption)

Reprinted with permission from the *Diagnostic and Statistical Manual of Mental Disorders, Fourth Edition*. Copyright 1994 American Psychiatric Association, Washington, D.C.

and causes noticeable distress or significant impairment in functioning. The criteria for dependence also include those that indicate physiological dependence (tolerance and withdrawal), as well as a loss of control as evidenced by repeated unsuccessful attempts to quit or cut down.

The term "addiction" closely resembles the definition of "dependence" as found in the *DSM-IV*. This is because the definition of dependence implies that there has been some change in the way the brain is functioning, as evidenced by the development of tolerance and withdrawal symptoms and by loss of control, which indicates the development of cravings.

But in an individual case, the distinction between abuse

and dependence is not always clear, because behavioral or descriptive criteria are imprecise. For practical purposes, we can say that people who meet the criteria for the abuse of a substance are at high risk for developing addiction or for already having the brain dysfunction that constitutes dependence or addiction.

For the clinician, distinguishing abuse from dependence is difficult but has important implications for predicting the course and prognosis of an individual's case. Dependence implies that biologically based addiction has occurred with the associated changes in brain functioning. If it were possible to measure this brain dysfunction with a scan or a test, the determination would be easy. But we can't do that, so we infer the diagnosis from behavior and history.

The philosophy of successful addiction treatment is based on the idea of complete abstinence from all mood-altering chemicals. This approach is the result of years of experience on the part of clinicians and of those with long-term recovery in programs such as Alcoholics Anonymous. But now and then a study is done revealing that a number of people who have gone through treatment for "alcoholism" have returned, apparently successfully, to social drinking. It may be that what was felt to be alcoholism was actually alcohol abuse and was not yet associated with the brain changes that occur in alcohol dependence. Until the distinction between alcohol abuse and dependence can be made with certainty, it would seem prudent to recommend total abstinence.

The criteria for diagnosing abuse or dependence are based on a look at the consequences that have occurred. But since the nature and degree of the consequences caused by the use of the substance depend to a large extent on what individuals are doing while intoxicated, it is also important to consider the entire context of their lives. For example, it can be difficult to identify any negative consequences of drinking (such as DUI arrests or loss of jobs) in a housewife who does all of her drinking at home alone. This is one of the reasons why alcoholism in women has been underrecognized. But a close look at the quality of such a person's relationships and achievements in the context of her social setting can often clarify the picture.

The stage of life someone is in is also important to consider. Regarding alcohol, for instance, it is not uncommon for young people who drink socially to go through a brief period of time when alcohol is abused for its intoxicating qualities. Sooner or later, however, some type of negative consequence will occur. It might be a bad hangover or an episode of embarrassing behavior. At that point most people will correctly identify the drinking as having caused the negative consequence and will modify their behavior. Some, however, continue to drink despite increasingly negative consequences—and this is addiction.

The prevailing culture is another factor. In a culture where daily social drinking is acceptable, the fact that someone is drinking regularly is less important. On the other hand, in cultures where drinking is highly frowned upon, even occasional alcohol use might be a concern. Smoking is another example. It has been said that as the prohibitions against smoking have increased, the characteristics of smokers have changed. Those who continue to smoke have a stronger addiction to nicotine, and are less able to use the methods for quitting that have worked for others. So a smoker in the late 1990s in the United States might be much more likely to have severe addiction than a smoker in the early 1950s.

Let's look at how use of a substance gradually progresses from social use to abuse to dependence (addiction). Some people never use an addictive substance. Others, who suffer minor consequences such as a hangover or an upset stomach, limit and control use of the substance. "Social drinkers" or "casual users" use the substance periodically, and some will continue to do so indefinitely if it does not cause much in the way of uncomfortable consequences. They are able to maintain control.

But some people, in continuing to use a substance, will escalate the amount and start to experience more negative consequences. Often this is the point at which the substance begins to be used more for its pharmacological effects—as a sedative or tranquilizer, for example. This "hazardous use" might lead to substantial consequences, and in some cases the person will recognize the problem and begin to abstain from the substance, therefore regaining control. Sometimes people go through a period of abusing substances during stressful periods in their lives. They might experience some fairly severe consequences, such as alcohol-related motor vehicle accidents, other legal charges, or behavioral problems related to intoxication. Some of these people will be able to recognize that using the substance is causing more trouble than it's worth. Control will be regained, and they will begin to abstain.

But some will continue using regularly despite repeated and increasingly severe consequences, exercising no control over the use of the substance. At this point in the continuum, dependence, not just abuse, is present. This is addiction. The continued use of the substance becomes the focal point of life. And when that change occurs, even when it is very subtle, all other aspects of life—relationships, jobs, responsibilities, goals—become less important than the addiction. It is not uncommon for an addict to lose everything before entering treatment. Incarceration or even death may occur before the addict has the chance to enter treatment.

When we think about the continuum from experimentation and casual use on to abuse and dependence, it is important to recognize that some people are probably genetically predisposed to developing dependence and also that the "addictiveness" of a substance will affect the rate at which loss of control and subsequent abuse and dependence occur.

These factors—genetic traits and the addictiveness of the substance—interact with each other in the development of addiction in an individual. People who come from families where there is a great deal of alcoholism and addiction may progress more quickly to dependence and addiction, even with substances that are less highly addictive for others. For those people, even social drinking may be hazardous. With highly addictive substances such as heroin and crack cocaine, genetics may be less important, and users may have little opportunity to experience negative consequences and to retreat from casual use before addiction occurs. So, with these substances, even experimentation can be dangerous.

## Is Addiction a Disease or a Moral Problem?

Most of us have grown up valuing self-control, sober judgment, and self-reliance. We look at addiction as a disgrace— something to be ashamed of. It represents lack of character and moral failure. We look at addicts as people who are untrustworthy, unreliable, irresponsible, and self-centered. Many religions view alcoholism and drug addiction as sinful. Ridding yourself of addiction, according to this line of thinking, involves realizing that you have a problem, repenting, and moving on in your life with renewed self-determination and responsibility.

On the other hand, addiction treatment centers teach addicts and their families the disease concept of addiction, which views alcoholism and addiction as a complex physical and psychological disorder. Addicts and alcoholics are felt to be sick and in need of treatment and understanding. Addiction is viewed as a chronic, relapsing, and potentially fatal disorder that can be treated if the proper conditions are met. Addiction professionals employ therapeutic techniques to deal with denial, research is done on medications that reduce cravings, and various therapeutic models such as cognitive-behavioral therapy are put forth as solutions.

These two positions—the moral model and the disease concept—are fairly divergent. But once again, like most things that have to do with addiction, both positions are too simplistic to capture the entire nature of addiction. Neither position is wrong, but neither is completely right.

Addiction *is* a brain disorder that some people are more prone to develop because of genetic, psychological, or environmental risk factors. *But* it does take an act of will—many acts of will, in fact—to get down the road far enough for the brain disorder of addiction to develop. Does this mean that people who develop addiction have only themselves to blame? No, I don't believe so. Life is so complex and has so many unforeseen risks that it makes no sense to place blame on the alcoholic or addict.

On the other hand, if you have an addiction it is still your responsibility to do something about it. It is around this issue of responsibility that the moral model of addiction and the disease concept of addiction come together. As I have lamented in many a treatment team meeting, "You can lead a horse to water, but you can't make him *not* drink."

Another way of looking at addiction is to think of it as a disorder of will. When the addiction sets in, your will is taken over by the need to use the drug—sometimes not completely, but enough so that you end up drinking or using a drug more often or in a greater quantity than you expected to. And as a result, your priorities change. The need to drink or use drugs takes precedence and leads to all kinds of dishonest, self-centered, and irresponsible behaviors. All too often the end result is incarceration, brain damage, or death. But if you take even the smallest step in the direction of sobriety and recovery, then you can take advantage of the therapies and treatments offered for the disease of addiction. This idea— taking the responsibility for one small step towards sobriety— is basic to recovery, and is reflected in the Alcoholics Anonymous slogan "Just for today."

In my opinion, the best way to approach addiction is to look at it as a brain disorder that can't be separated from morality and personal responsibility. You may not have asked for the addiction, but you must ask for help to recover, and you must be willing to accept responsibility for your choices.

# 2. Who Gets Addicted and How?

If you are struggling with addiction, you probably did not intend for it to happen. People who begin using mood-altering substances usually have a number of reasons for doing so.

Most of the patients that I have treated tell me that they first used an addictive substance in their midteens. They typically report that they began drinking beer with friends on weekends at about the age of fifteen or sixteen. But, after a while, things would change. Future "social drinkers" find the effect of the beer mildly interesting, but not worth the effort if it makes them sick or gets them into trouble. But the future alcoholic or addict often reacts to the first use of a mood-altering drug with a sense of having finally found a way to feel "normal." We now know that there are probably genetic differences in the brains of alcoholics and addicts that cause them to have this exaggerated reaction.

When I was in medical school, a professor once suggested that a way to determine whether a patient was likely to be alcoholic was to see whether the person could remember his or her first drink. I have routinely asked this when taking histories, and I find that in many cases they can. Alcoholics and addicts (who often start with alcohol) are likely to remember their first drink as a distinctly pleasurable experience. "I finally felt like I could fit in and socialize" is a statement I hear frequently. People say that the first time they used marijuana they were able to feel relief from chronic anxiety or that the first time they used stimulants they got relief from chronic depression.

Naturally such a positive experience will probably be repeated. If you find that drinking or using drugs helps you to solve a problem such as shyness, anxiety, or depression, then it is likely that you will start to look for opportunities to obtain and use alcohol and drugs. It is this initial effect that provides the motivation for the continuing use of a substance.

People who work with alcohol and drug abuse prevention try to influence young people not to begin experimenting with drugs for just this reason. They feel that focusing later efforts at the treatment stage is like closing the barn door after the horse gets out. We do know that there are many people who come from families with a strong history of addiction who decide never to try alcohol or drugs. Those people manage eventually to work out their emotional problems, finding other ways of coping besides using a mood-altering drug. But once a vulnerable person has used alcohol or another mood-altering drug, a powerful learning effect takes place, especially if the person is young and not yet mature.

### Factors Influencing Early Use

Why would you decide to experiment with drugs and alcohol at all? This decision depends to a large extent on the type of family and community that you come from. If you are raised in a society with strict taboos against the use of mood-altering drugs, as in Islamic culture, for example, the opportunity to experiment might never arise, and therefore addiction would not be an issue.

But in middle-class America, experimentation with drugs and alcohol is quite common in the teen and young adult years. If you have watched your parents have a drink in the afternoon to wind down, then you get the message that using alcohol or drugs in order to feel better is acceptable—at least within certain limits. Television and movies often portray characters who drink, and there is a constant push, through advertising, for us to "grab all the gusto" or celebrate "Miller time." So you may have first used simply because you wanted to grow up faster or to conform.

## Availability

The substance that someone starts experimenting with is usually what is available at that time. If you were raised in the fifties and early sixties, you may never have encountered any illicit drugs at all in high school or even in college. Unless you had access to marijuana, for example, there would be no opportunity to try it. But by the mid-to-late sixties, all types of drugs were readily available on college campuses, and by the eighties even a grade-school child could obtain drugs fairly easily.

"Gateway drugs" open the door to further experimentation. Caffeine and nicotine, for example, are gateway drugs. Once you have the initial experience of changing your mood with a substance, you're probably less resistant to using something else. Smoking and drinking coffee, then, might be a gateway to using alcohol. Alcohol might be a gateway to trying marijuana, which is a gateway to trying something like LSD or cocaine, and so on.

## Peer Pressure

Peer pressure is often the impetus for someone to begin experimenting with alcohol and drugs. People vary in the degree to which they will respond to such pressure. In an interesting psychology experiment years ago, researchers recruited college students who were told that visual perception was being studied. Each student was placed in a room with a group of other people. Slides were shown of parallel lines, and the group was asked to say which line was longest, those other than the student having been secretly instructed to answer incorrectly each time. The student was subjected to a dilemma—it was obvious which line was longest, but the group said something different. A majority of the student subjects went along with the group, even though they admitted later that they knew the answer was wrong.

The need to conform with the group is very strong, especially for young people. But when a person's family is supportive and intact and there are opportunities to socialize and participate in rewarding activities, the pressure to use drugs or drink has less effect.

### Family Disruption

One reason that future alcoholics and addicts are vulnerable to peer pressure may be that they already have problems with self-esteem or have difficulties at home. If you are an alcoholic or drug addict, it is quite likely that someone in your family has had problems with addiction. This is because there are genetic factors in the development of addiction. Even if the family member is a grandparent, aunt, or uncle, it's highly likely that some damage has been done to the structure of your extended family that affected your upbringing. The net result of growing up in such a family is that you are not provided with a stable basis for help in developing self-esteem and an individual identity. This can make you more vulnerable to peer pressure, and, in turn, lead you to engage in certain behaviors even though you can see the resulting problems in your family. Such a situation is ironic but not uncommon.

### Psychological Trauma

You may have an even more compelling reason to experiment with drugs and alcohol. You may be one of the large number of alcoholics and addicts who have a history of being abused or neglected as a child. You may actually be living in an abusive situation at the time that you choose to experiment, and the relief that you get from painful feelings is a powerful reinforcer. People in this situation have a difficult time with early recovery, because the feelings start to surface after a short period of abstinence.

If this was your situation, and you are in recovery, you should find a competent psychologist or psychiatrist who can help you deal with these feelings rather than trying to cover them up by getting high.

### How Addictions Develop

In chapter 1, we saw that people can be said to be addicted when they lose control over the use of a substance and continue that behavior despite negative consequences. In such a case, using the substance takes precedence over all other goals and responsibilities in the person's life, often to the point of incarceration or death. We've also seen that not everybody who drinks or uses drugs ends up losing control. So how is it that some people become addicted and some don't?

Because addiction is a multifaceted problem with many aspects, the answer to this question is simply, "Well, it depends . . ." So let's see if we can get a grip on how addictions develop.

One way of thinking about addiction is to compare it to an infectious disease, like the flu. At the beginning of an outbreak of the flu, the virus is introduced into the population by one person. Since the flu is spread by airborne contact—sneezing and coughing—it begins to spread quickly. But does everyone who is exposed to the virus get the flu? No. Does everyone who experiments with an addictive substance become an addict? No.

Let's look at our comparison with the flu from an epidemiological standpoint. A number of factors are in play, and these can be put into three groups: host, environmental, and agent.

*Host Factors*

Some people inherit a tendency to develop addiction. We will examine the genetics of addiction in more detail later on in this chapter.

Psychological factors may also increase or decrease an individual's vulnerability to becoming addicted. People with psychiatric disorders such as clinical depression or anxiety have a higher risk of developing addiction. People who come from disrupted homes or who have been abused are also more prone to develop addiction.

Some personality factors may make a person more likely to experiment or to use. Risk takers, people with poor impulse control or low stress tolerance, and people who have difficulty learning from negative consequences are at increased risk.

*Environmental Factors*

Environmental factors might include the cultural acceptance of social use of the substance, the availability of a substance in the community, the degree of criminality associated with use of the substance, and so on. Community prevention and education programs aim at modifying the environmental aspect of the spread of addiction.

An example of the importance of environmental factors is seen in the rise of crack cocaine addiction in the late 1980s. Powder cocaine, which is used intranasally (being snorted) was readily available in the early 1980s, but was fairly expensive. Extracting the cocaine base from the powder form of the drug, called free-basing, allowed for intravenous and inhalation use—methods that intensified the high—but was a somewhat involved and dangerous chemical process requiring the use of highly flammable chemicals. (The actor Richard Pryor was severely burned while free-basing.) Some clever but diabolical individual discovered, however, that you could take powder cocaine, dissolve and dilute it, mix it with common household chemicals, and cook it in the microwave to produce a crystalline form of cocaine called "rock" or "crack" cocaine that could be smoked in a pipe for an immediate and intense, although brief, high. This was a marketing coup for the drug cartels, because someone could take a kilogram of cocaine and produce mountains of cocaine rocks that could be sold very cheaply. The going price for a rock in some urban locations dropped below a dollar, opening the market to younger and less affluent users. Crack rocks were also much easier to conceal and transport than bulkier drugs like marijuana. The use of crack spread like wildfire, and so, unfortunately, did the intense addiction that it causes.

### Agent Factors

Agent factors, which relate to the specific characteristics of the disease-causing entity, are important in addiction, involving the addictiveness of the substance itself. Addictiveness is an estimate of a substance's tendency to be abused and its ability to result in compulsive use regardless of other factors. As we will see later, all classes of addictive substances that have been studied so far interact with a certain part of the brain, but some are more potent than others in their effects on that organ.

The route of administration of a particular substance is also an important agent factor. In general, the oral form of a drug is less addictive than the intravenous form, which is less addictive than the inhaled form. This has to do with the speed at which the drug reaches the brain. When drugs are taken orally, they can take up to an hour or more to peak in the brain circulation. Drugs taken intravenously peak in the brain circulation within minutes, inhaled drugs within seconds. The rate at which the drug enters the brain contributes to the risk of an addiction developing. Studies have shown that the strength of the learning effect on primitive parts of the brain correlates more closely with the rate at which the drug's concentration increases than it does with the total concentration at its peak.

When we look at all these factors—host, environment, and agent—we can see how they come together in a particular situation to determine whether an individual will develop addiction. Some examples follow.

Tom, Sr., had grown up in an alcoholic family. His father, his father's father, and all his uncles on his father's side were alcoholic. When Tom was a child, he decided that he would never, ever drink alcohol. He remained a teetotaller all his life. He was successful and prominent in his community and church. His son, Tommy, also did not drink while living at home. However, when Tommy went to college, he drank beer for the first time at a fraternity party. That night he became extremely intoxicated, and could not remember anything after the first one or two beers. He began to drink on weekends and was soon drinking daily. He was expelled from college when his grades dropped to D's and F's.

Tommy's roommate, Bob, had grown up in a family that had no alcoholics except for one distant cousin. His parents drank socially, and never to excess. Bob first drank some in high school with friends, and continued to drink at frat parties in college. At one point, while having problems with a girlfriend, he drank heavily for a while, but after getting sick at a party he cut back on his use. He continues to drink socially and only occasionally, without serious consequences.

Tommy and Bob were both exposed to alcohol in an environment that encouraged drinking. However, Tommy had inherited a genetic vulnerability to alcoholism that was not apparent in his father because his father never allowed himself to be exposed to alcohol. Whereas Bob was able to moderate his use of alcohol after experiencing some unpleasant consequences, Tommy was not.

Angela began drinking at thirteen, and shortly after that began using marijuana whenever it was available to her. By the time she dropped out of high school, she was using drugs on a daily basis, including marijuana, pain pills, tranquilizers, LSD, and powder cocaine. She came from a disturbed home and was abused and neglected as a child by her drug-addicted mother and various stepfathers. By the time she was twenty-five, she was using crack cocaine almost exclusively, because it gave her the most intense high. She was living on the streets and supporting herself through prostitution.

Tanya came from a stable working-class home; she was a good student and active in her church youth group. No one in her family had ever had problems with alcohol or drugs. She did not drink or smoke at all while she was in high school. After graduating from junior college and getting a secretarial job, she began going out with friends, and drank a little at parties. A man she was dating encouraged her to try some crack cocaine, assuring her that she wouldn't get hooked if she used it only occasionally. However, within six months Tanya was using as much crack as she could get three or four times a week. She had lost her job and was living on the street supporting herself through prostitution.

Angela and Tanya both ended up with tragic lifestyles that centered around the addiction to crack cocaine. But they came from very different backgrounds. In Angela's case, crack eventually took over as her drug of choice, but she had both psychological and genetic factors that favored her developing an addiction. While Tanya had no psychological or genetic factors to push her into addiction, she became trapped by a very addictive substance.

In both of the preceding examples, the environment was favorable for drinking or using drugs. In Tommy's case, host factors were critical—he inherited the risk of alcoholism from his father, even though his father never drank. In Angela's case, host factors included her history of severe abuse, which led her to learn to use chemicals to affect her mood. But in Tanya's case, there were very few host factors. What got her in trouble was an agent factor—the strong addictive nature of crack cocaine.

## The Genetics of Addiction

Although we know that the risk for alcoholism runs in some families, it is not clear exactly what genes cause the increased risk. (There is good evidence that several genes are involved.)

Most of the genetic studies that have been done on addiction have dealt with alcoholism, but there is growing evidence that many of the basic principles apply to other drugs as well. In fact, statistical analysis shows that if you have relatives with drug dependence, you are at substantially increased risk of becoming addicted to any drug, including alcohol.

But it seems as though the risk is higher pertaining to the specific drug that your relatives are addicted to. If they are alcoholic, your risk of becoming alcoholic increases; if they are addicted to opiates, you are at increased risk for that addiction. The same seems true for marijuana, cocaine, and nicotine.

Whenever we wonder if a condition is inherited, we have to ask ourselves whether the trait that we see in both parent and child is caused by transmission through the genes or by some common factor in the environment. For example, how do we know whether a child who loves music and is talented in that field inherited the characteristic or is just benefiting from growing up in surroundings where music is appreciated?

Researchers approach this question by looking for cases of children who have been adopted, or, even better for purposes of investigation, identical twins who were separated at birth and have been raised in different families. Some countries, such as Denmark, have maintained registries of twins and of adoptions for many years, so that the records are available for research. When these are analyzed regarding the subject of addiction, some patterns begin to emerge.

Studies of twins are especially useful. Geneticists classify identical twins as monozygotic, meaning that they developed from one egg, and fraternal twins as dizygotic, meaning that they came from two different eggs (a zygote is a fertilized egg). Identical twins have 100 percent of the same genes and fraternal twins about 50 percent of the same genes. When twins exhibit the same trait, it is called concordance.

The risk of addiction regardless of family history is about one in ten. If an identical twin is alcoholic, there is more than a 50 percent chance that the other twin will be alcoholic, even if they are reared apart. On the other hand, fraternal twins reared apart have about the same risk of developing alcoholism as other siblings of alcoholics—about a one-in-four risk. The concordance rates, therefore, are about 50 percent for monozygotes and about 25 percent for dizygotes, indicating that genes play an important role in addiction. That identical twins don't have a 100 percent concordance rate as they would for physical traits such as eye color shows that nongenetic factors are also important.

Adoption studies help us to sort out genetic factors from environmental ones. Children whose biological parents were alcoholic are far more likely than others to become alcoholic even if their adoptive parents are not alcoholic. In fact, the biological child of an alcoholic parent is three to five times more likely to be alcoholic than the biological child of nonalcoholic parents, even in nonalcoholic families that are considered well-adjusted and functional.

It can be shown by statistical means that inheritance accounts for about 50 percent of the risk of an individual becoming alcoholic. Some other traits, such as impulsiveness, aggressiveness, and antisocial tendencies, are also likely to be passed down from the biological parents—regardless of the traits of the adoptive parents. These traits contribute to the risk for addiction but appear to function independently of the basic genetic flaw that puts relatives of alcoholics and addicts at risk for addiction.

One clever way to study the genetics of addiction is to use animal models. A group of researchers in the 1970s began selectively breeding lab rats who appeared to enjoy water spiked with alcohol. Gradually, two groups of rats were bred: "P" rats (alcohol-preferring) and "NP" rats (alcohol nonpreferring). The "P" rats not only bred true but also developed many behaviors reminiscent of a human alcoholic. For example, they would consistently opt for spiked water in place of some of their rat chow, and they would go on binges, developing blood alcohol levels of up to four times what the legal driving limit would be for humans. This study was important because it helped to prove that genetic factors *alone*—regardless of the environment—could lead to alcoholism.

### Type I and Type II Alcoholics

Early family studies identified two broad categories of alcoholics, who differed in the pattern of inheritance. C. Robert Cloniger of Washington University in St. Louis developed this concept when he described two clinically identifiable subgroups of alcoholics, which he termed Type I and Type II. In the 1980s diagnostic classifications reflected this dichotomy; alcohol dependence was divided into "continuous" and "episodic" types. Even though we don't fully understand the genetic traits that go into this grouping, it has proven to be reliable.

Type I alcoholics tend to have mothers who are alcoholic, to have the onset of alcoholic drinking in their thirties or forties, to be anxious, rigid, and emotionally dependent, and to experience loss of control of the use of alcohol only after several decades of use. These alcoholics tend to engage in binge drinking rather than continuous drinking and also to be more reactive to environmental factors, which is why the term "milieu limited" is used to describe them.

Type II alcoholics tend to have fathers who are alcoholic,

to have the onset of alcoholic drinking before age twenty-five, and to have problems with conduct, aggression, and impulsiveness and an inclination for novelty-seeking behaviors. These alcoholics tend to be continuous drinkers who have a great deal of difficulty remaining abstinent for any prolonged length of time, to develop alcoholic drinking patterns very quickly after the onset of alcohol use, and to seem less affected by their environments. Because this group appears to be almost exclusively male, with the risk transmitted through fathers, it is termed "male limited."

It has also been shown that there are physiological differences between these two groups. For example, their brain waves differ under various conditions, and they differ consistently in personality traits and temperament (table 2.1).

### Trait Markers

We know, then, that you are much more likely to develop an addiction if there's addiction in your family. But what exactly is inherited that causes this to occur? Answering that has been difficult indeed. One way of doing research

**Table 2.1.**

|  | Type I | Type II |
| --- | --- | --- |
| Onset of alcoholism | after age twenty-five | before age twenty-five |
| Fighting, arrests | infrequent | frequent |
| Feelings of guilt, apprehension | frequent | infrequent |
| Novelty-seeking behavior | infrequent | frequent |
| Introversion | frequent | infrequent |
| Alcoholic parent | mother | father |
| Drinking pattern | episodic | continuous |
| Effect of milieu | significant | insignificant |

is to look for trait markers, which are traits that are found to be strongly associated with the condition being studied. These traits *might* be related in some way to that condition, although they might just be linked by some other coincidental factor.

When we study relatives of alcoholics and of nonalcoholics, some differences begin to emerge, and these appear to be trait markers for alcoholism. One is called the "low response factor." Sons of alcoholics, when given a measured dose of alcohol, will have much less of a behavioral response than sons of nonalcoholics. In fact, if we look closely at the statistics, this trait probably accounts to a large degree for the inheritance of the addiction to alcohol. Having a blunted response to the intoxicating effects of alcohol probably allows a person to drink more and also more often, especially at an early age. It is thought to increase the risk of developing an addiction to alcohol because it allows for more prolonged exposure of the brain to the addicting drug.

Another difference between sons of alcoholics and sons of nonalcoholics is seen when we measure body sway after a dose of alcohol. To do this, a person is given a dose of alcohol and then told to stand still, feet together and hands at the side. The number of degrees off the vertical that the person's body sways is then measured. If the family history is negative for alcoholism, there is much more body sway than if the family history is positive. What this means is that people with a genetic risk for alcoholism don't seem to have as much impairment in motor functioning when they drink the same amount of alcohol. Again, this is probably important in the development of alcoholism because it affects how the person feels and functions while drinking. It's as though people who have alcoholism in the family are somehow better suited—at first—to tolerate the short-term effects of drinking. They are less likely to have a negative experience early on and probably more likely to continue drinking, which will lead eventually to alcohol dependence.

Some other traits that sons of alcoholic fathers have include differences found on a brain wave test (electroencephalogram, or EEG) and a blunting of the brain's electrical response to a specific stimulus (event-related potential, or ERP).

A genetic trait that appears to actually protect people from developing alcoholism involves a metabolizing enzyme. When alcohol is consumed, the body breaks it down into a compound called acetaldehyde, which is then further broken down and eliminated from the body. The enzyme called alcohol dehydrogenase is necessary to break down the acetaldehyde. However, many people lack a certain form of the enzyme. They build up large amounts of acetaldehyde in their system, which causes them to feel ill, with flushing, rapid heartbeat, and burning in the stomach. Asians commonly have this trait. For those people, drinking alcohol is a very unpleasant experience and not likely to be repeated. A similar phenomenon is exploited when we use the drug disulfiram (Antabuse), which disables the enzyme. Someone who drinks while taking disulfiram will become physically ill, so that the drug can be used as a deterrent.

So we can see that there are measurable differences between people with family histories of alcoholism and those without. But what is the mechanism that causes people with such histories to become addicted?

As we will learn in the next chapter, all addictive drugs interact in one way or another with a certain part of the brain commonly referred to as the "pleasure center." Many researchers are focusing on this part of the brain in alcoholics and in nonalcoholics, trying to find some type of clearly inherited differences. This is, of course, a daunting task. It sometimes seems as though the more we learn, the more we realize how complicated the brain is. But we do know a few things.

Endorphins are naturally occurring opiates that are found in tiny amounts in specific parts of the brain. They play a role in pain modulation as well as in the regulation of mood states. Alcohol's addictive properties appear to involve a mechanism most simply described as the brain getting hooked on its own opiates. This explains why alcoholics and their relatives have an exaggerated secretion of endorphins which can be measured in the bloodstream, and why an opiate-blocking drug such as naltrexone is an effective aid for treating alcoholism in some people. If you have a family history of alcoholism, your body may actually react to alcohol as strongly as it would to a drug like morphine.

This abnormal reaction has been studied statistically through measurement of the circulating blood levels of a compound known as ß-endorphin. After a person is exposed to alcohol, levels of ß-endorphin tend to rise in those with a family history of alcoholism but not in those with no such history. (This effect is seen when large groups are analyzed, but cannot as yet be used to diagnose the risk of alcoholism in an individual.)

A great deal of research is being done on the effectiveness of opiate-blocking drugs like naltrexone (Revia, Trexan) in the treatment of alcoholism. These drugs blunt the activity of opiate receptors in the brain. In other words, they prevent the brain from producing a euphoric response to opiates. In alcoholics, naltrexone has been shown to increase periods of abstinence and decrease the severity of relapses.

Another chemical thought to be important in the brain's response to addictive substances is dopamine. Dopamine is one of numerous chemicals that communicate messages between nerve cells. Most of the nerve cells in the pleasure center of the brain are activated when there is increased brain activity of dopamine. Researchers are examining the chemical receptors that allow nerve cells to respond to dopamine. It appears that some people from alcoholic families tend to have defects in these receptors.

This may mean that for the people with a genetic risk of alcoholism the pleasure center doesn't work just right. The experience of being intoxicated provides a sense of well-being that might otherwise be absent. The brain quickly learns that it can feel "normal" when the substance is present, and so there is strong motivation for an individual to use alcohol again and again. Fortunately, the majority of people who get sober and stay in recovery do *not* give up a sense of well-being. In fact, many recovering people say that although they felt good drinking or doing drugs at first, they have never felt better psychologically than they do in recovery.

Mechanisms causing a unique response to an addictive drug are probably also in play with marijuana, cocaine, heroin, and other drugs. The risk of becoming addicted to one of these drugs is higher for those with others in the family who are addicted than it is in the general population.

## Psychological and Behavioral Factors

If genetics accounts for better than 50 percent of the risk, what accounts for the remaining percentage? A lot of things do. Going back to our infectious model, comparison of addiction and infectious disease, we can see that there are environmental factors such as the availability of the drug and the permissiveness of the culture, as well as agent factors such as the addictiveness of the substance.

But psychological factors play an enormous role in the development of addiction. Some of these factors, as we've seen, have a genetic basis. Traits such as aggressiveness, impulsiveness, and antisocial tendencies tend to run in families independently of addiction. They put people at risk for using alcohol and drugs, especially at a young age. And the only way to develop an addiction is to be exposed to the drug in the first place.

Beyond these traits, though, lie other psychological factors that promote the development of addiction. Remember that each of these drugs stimulates the pleasure center of the brain, and they all affect mood. Being able to change one's mood instantly is tempting to a person plagued with chronic depression or anxiety. Medical treatment of depression and anxiety may not be completely effective for everyone, and psychotherapy is time consuming and difficult. Many people who are depressed or anxious don't have ready access to psychiatric services, and they come to feel that the use of alcohol or drugs as a coping mechanism is a useful compromise in the short term.

A history of psychological trauma also puts a person at risk for addiction. Posttraumatic stress disorder, or PTSD, is a reactive state that occurs after a severe, life-threatening trauma, and we know that people with PTSD are at increased risk of addiction. We saw this clearly illustrated during the years of the war in Vietnam. Many returning servicemen had begun using alcohol, marijuana, or heroin while overseas as a way to tolerate the severe stress of combat. Although many veterans quit alcohol or drugs after coming home, a number continued to suffer chronic anxiety and tension as a reaction to their combat experiences. And many developed addiction as a result, even though they were no longer in a combat setting.

One problem with PTSD is that the physiological reaction to the trauma does not subside with time. When confronted with a sudden life-or-death situation, the body reacts by secreting adrenaline and gearing up to either defend itself or run. We call this the "fight or flight" reaction; it is usually followed by a brief emotional collapse and then quick recuperation from the experience. But in those with PTSD it's as though this reaction cannot be turned off. The person is jittery, fearful, and hyperalert. Sleep is disrupted, sometimes by vivid nightmares, and the individual experiences a general emotional numbing towards other people and situations. Sometimes the traumatic event seems to occur over and over again, like an instant replay, even while the person is awake; these flashbacks are painful and isolating. If the traumatic situation is ongoing, or the reaction to it persists for a long time, depression eventually sets in. Mood-altering drugs override the brain's emotional centers, and people with PTSD often discover that drinking, smoking marijuana, or using other types of drugs is an effective way to temporarily change mood and get some respite from their misery. Unfortunately, addiction often follows, and even this way of managing painful feelings no longer helps but only makes things worse.

The disorder is overrepresented in people with addiction. It is not confined just to combat veterans, but is found as well in people who have suffered abuse or have been victims of crime, severe accidents, or natural disasters. Stopping the use of the alcohol or drugs means that the symptoms and painful feelings must be dealt with in another way. If the problems are ignored, relapse is a potential problem.

Another class of psychological problems that tends to promote addiction is the personality disorders. A personality disorder is a mode of reacting to life's stresses that is usually fixed in place by problems that occurred early in a person's life. It's a stable pattern of maladjustment. People with personality disorders are "one-tool carpenters." They have a limited range of responses to problems and often find themselves in conflict with other people or with the world.

Those with personality disorders frequently lack insight into their own behavior, tending to see their problems as being caused by their situation or by someone else. As a result, they have a hard time making lasting adaptations to new situations. Such people find it difficult to carry out the changes necessary to recover from addiction, but many can do so over time.

Borderline personality disorder is believed to arise from a combination of genetic and environmental factors. Most people with borderline personality disorder were severely abused, often sexually, as children. The abused child develops an early fixation that provides a way for him or her to cope unconsciously with overwhelming anxiety. The fixation is useful for that purpose, but it severely cripples a person in the development of mature relationships, the handling of stress and conflict, and the creation of a consistent personal identity. Alcohol or drug abuse of an on-again, off-again nature is common in people with this disorder, and some go on to become addicted.

Antisocial personality disorder also appears to have roots in childhood development, but there is evidence that vulnerability to this disorder is passed along in families as well. In fact, a link may exist between Type II alcoholism and antisocial personality, and there also seems to be some overlap with attention deficit disorder. People with antisocial personality disorder are deficient in their ability to relate to other people in a mutual fashion, seeming to be able to relate only to the extent that others meet their immediate needs. They also have difficulty with conduct, ethics, and mores. They judge their own actions by utility ("Is this going to get me what I want?") rather than by morality ("Is this the right thing to do?"). They also seem to have difficulty learning from painful experience, which puts them at tremendous risk for addiction since they are unlikely to avoid a mood-altering substance that gives immediate gratification even if they have had a bad experience with it in the past.

Attention deficit disorder is commonly known as hyperactivity. It is diagnosed in children, but follow-up studies have shown that as many as 40 percent of people diagnosed with the disorder do not outgrow the problem. Those with attention deficit disorder have difficulty sustaining a train of thought for as long as is necessary to complete a task. Children with the disorder have trouble in school, are impulsive, and appear immature. We used to believe that hyperactivity was usually present, but now we know that a substantial number of children have a type of attention deficit disorder characterized by inattention. These children do not behave the way hyperactive kids do, but they have the same problems with sustaining attention.

Adults who had attention deficit disorder as children have an increased risk of developing alcohol or drug dependence.

They also have a tendency toward underachievement and low self-esteem. Attention deficit disorder is often treated with drugs from the amphetamine family. Sometimes a person with unrecognized or untreated attention deficit disorder will discover that the stimulants available on the street are effective in reversing the symptoms of impaired attention, and this begins a process that often leads to addiction. Nicotine also seems to have a beneficial effect, and it's thought that many hard-core smokers are actually people with this disorder who find it difficult to function without cigarettes and therefore have a hard time quitting.

Biologically based brain disorders include major depression, panic and anxiety disorders, schizophrenia, and bipolar disorder (manic-depression). We know that all of the biologically based brain disorders increase the risk that a person will develop addiction. Having one of these disorders is a powerful host factor in the risk for addiction. Mood-altering drugs are often fairly effective at first in managing the symptoms of these disorders, which are painful and disruptive.

The concept of an "addictive personality" has been quite popular. According to this idea, there are people who, because of their personalities, engage in excessive behavior with a given drug or activity. There is no scientific basis for this assumption. As we have seen, there appears to be an inherited risk for addiction that runs in families, but it only accounts for about half the risk, and does not correlate with any particular personality characteristics. The remaining proportion of risk can be attributed to a wide variety of disorders, as well as to social and cultural factors. However, the concept of an "addictive personality" just won't die despite reams of research. I have worked with a lot of people with addiction, and my hunch is that this concept lives on because it provides some with a ready excuse for continuing addictive behaviors and not taking responsibility for recovery, which is difficult to do.

# 3. The Addicted Brain

Only within the last several decades have we begun to understand why a person will use a substance compulsively, regardless of the consequences, even to the point of death. The key to understanding this puzzling behavior lies in a series of discoveries made over the last forty years. In the 1950s it was learned that if a certain part of the brain is electrically stimulated, an intensely pleasurable sensation occurs. In the 1960s researchers began to find receptors in the brain for opiate-like substances. Later in that decade the discovery was made that the brain produces opiate-like substances (endorphins), which explained the presence of the opiate receptors.

## The Pleasure Center

As addiction has been studied in the past couple of decades, we have found that *alcohol and every major class of drugs of abuse* interact with the same part of the brain in one fashion or another. This part of the brain is the same one that produces the intensely pleasurable reaction to electrical stimulation that was noted in the 1950s. It is located in the lower central portion of the brain, the part that regulates automatic functions such as breathing and appetite. It is connected to the relay centers of the brain that include the thalamus and hypothalamus, as well as to higher parts of the brain such as the cortex, where most of our learning and reasoning take place. This part of the brain is called the ventral tegmentum and is part of a circuit known as the medial forebrain bundle. It includes tracts of nerve cells called the mesolimbic tracts.

The primary purpose of this part of the brain seems to be to produce a pleasurable sensation when it is stimulated and to make sure that the higher parts of the brain remember what the stimulation was so that it will be repeated. This area is intertwined with parts important in memory and learning and with those which control appetite and sexual desire (fig. 3.1).

The cells that make up this area are rich in the same neurotransmitters (see below) which regulate emotion, and their fibers extend to and interact with the structure of the brain that mediates emotional tone (the limbic system).

It has been consistently demonstrated that drugs with addictive properties are active in the ventral tegmentum. In fact, one way in which researchers study addictive drugs is to stimulate that area in the brain of an animal and then observe its behavior. If the animal is hooked up to electrodes that it can learn to stimulate by pressing a lever, it will press that lever over and over—even in lieu of food—until it falls out in exhaustion. A researcher who hooks the animal up to a tiny infusing device that delivers a drug can see whether the animal pushes the lever in the same manner. If the animal does push the lever, the indication is that the infused substance is

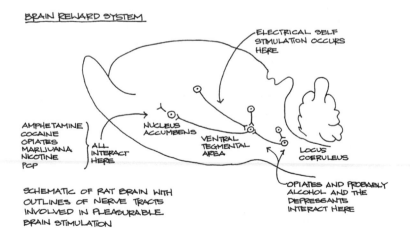

BRAIN REWARD SYSTEM

ELECTRICAL SELF STIMULATION OCCURS HERE

AMPHETAMINE COCAINE OPIATES MARIJUANA NICOTINE PCP

ALL INTERACT HERE

NUCLEUS ACCUMBENS

VENTRAL TEGMENTAL AREA

LOCUS COERULEUS

OPIATES AND PROBABLY ALCOHOL AND THE DEPRESSANTS INTERACT HERE

SCHEMATIC OF RAT BRAIN WITH OUTLINES OF NERVE TRACTS INVOLVED IN PLEASURABLE BRAIN STIMULATION

FIG. 3.1.Adapted from Wise, RA. Action of drugs of abuse on brain reward mechanisms. Pharmacol Biochem Behav 1980; 13 (suppl 1): 213–23. (*Substance Abuse: A Comprehensive Textbook.* 2nd. ed. Lowinson, Joyce H., M.D., et al., eds. Baltimore: Williams and Wilkins, 1992.)

stimulating that area of the brain. The frequency with which the animal pushes the lever also measures the potency of the drug in question—the more it pushes, the stronger the effect of the drug.

This response to all the known drugs of abuse is so consistent that use of the technique has become standard practice in the testing of new drugs for addictive potential. If a researcher infuses the drug and the animal goes on behaving normally, then the drug is probably not addictive.

### Neurotransmitters

Although a number of circuits with different neurotransmitters connect to and run through the ventral tegmentum, the main tracts use dopamine. Other important tracts use serotonin, norepinephrine, or endorphin. Let's look further at what neurotransmitters are and what they do.

Brain cells communicate messages via chemicals in the brain that are called neurotransmitters. Neurotransmitters are compounds that are secreted at the end of a nerve cell when it is electrically stimulated by another cell attached to it. They are secreted into a tiny gap between the cells, which is called a synapse (fig. 3.2). As they dissolve into the fluid within the

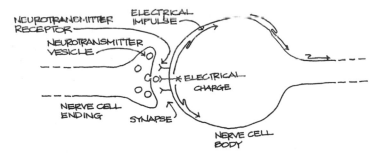

FIG. 3.2.

synapse, some of these molecules become bound to receptors. Receptors and neurotransmitters function in a lock-and-key fashion. The receptor is shaped precisely to fit the specific neurotransmitter it needs. Other chemicals will not bind at all, or might bind only loosely, producing a weaker signal.

Nerve cells generally produce only one kind of chemical. This is what allows messages to flow in tracts, which are laid out in a fashion similar to an electrical circuit within the brain. One of the most common neurotransmitters involved in emotions and behaviors is called serotonin, or 5-hydroxytryptamine.

The suffix "ergic" is attached to the name of the specific neurotransmitter so as to identify which type of nerve cell it is. Nerve cells that produce serotonin are called serotoninergic and those that secrete dopamine are called dopaminergic neurons. The producers of norepinephrine (a substance similar to adrenaline) are called adrenergic, and the ones that produce peptides, such as endorphins and others, are called peptidergic.

What starts out sounding like a fairly simple pattern—nerve cells communicating with each other in a specific chemical chain—is actually complicated. It might help to think of the brain as resembling an ecosystem. Years ago we thought of clinical depression as involving a lack either of serotonin or of norepinephrine, which leads to a chemical imbalance—kind of like tipping a seesaw. We know now that there are no fewer than fifteen different subtypes of serotonin receptors, some of which perform opposite functions, and the list is growing at the research labs. We also know that there are other chemicals involved in depression, perhaps farther "upstream" or "downstream," and that the nature of how these circuits work with one another can be influenced by other factors. So it's not a simple seesaw, after all.

Just as the loss of one species can change the environment of an entire forest or marsh, a change in the activity of just one neurotransmitter can have a cascade effect. As these tracts of nerve cells interact with each other, broad shifts occur within the chemical environment of the brain. Stimulation of one area by a specific drug might have a direct effect, as well as a number of secondary effects resulting from changes that occur in the system as a whole. This is important to remember when we try to understand the wide variety of behavioral and emotional changes associated with the use of and addiction to mood-altering drugs.

Neurotransmitters are released by nerve cells when the cell membrane receives an electrical charge. The cell membrane is a porous sac composed of specialized fats and tiny protein complexes. Ionized salts such as sodium, potassium, chloride, or calcium line the inside and outside of this membrane, and produce an electrical charge, much like that of a battery. Tiny channels that function like gates allow movement of these chemicals inside and outside of the cell, in response to interactions with chemicals, usually neurotransmitters. Once a neurotransmitter settles into its receptor, like a key fitting into a lock, these channels open and allow the ions to move. This changes the membrane's electrical charge, which moves in a wave-like fashion along the cell from the cell body to the axon, then to the nerve endings or synapses. Once this wave of electrical charge reaches the nerve ending at the synapse, a tiny packet of neurotransmitter is released into the synapse. This neurotransmitter then attaches to the body of the next cell in the chain, starting a chain reaction along the nerve tract.

The neurotransmitter in the synapse is deactivated in one of two ways. It is either taken back up into the nerve ending of the cell that released it—a process we call reuptake—or it is degraded by enzymes that are found in the synapse. If the neurotransmitter is not taken back up or degraded, the signal continues, as if someone were holding a finger down on a doorbell button.

Most of the drugs that are prescribed for psychiatric conditions such as depression or anxiety work indirectly, either by affecting the rate of reuptake of the neurotransmitter or by inhibiting its destruction by enzymes within the synapse. The nerve cell itself and the tract it belongs to continue functioning as they are supposed to, firing or shutting down appropriately, depending on the stimulus. On the other hand, mood-altering drugs—those with the potential to be addictive—often override this system by tricking the nerve cell into thinking it is being stimulated by a natural neurotransmitter.

### What Are Addictive Substances?

In chapter 4 we will discuss the major drugs of abuse, including alcohol. But first we are going to look at some general principles that apply to all addictive substances.

As we have seen, drugs that have the potential for addiction interact in one manner or another with a part of the brain known as the ventral tegmentum, or the pleasure center. We also know that all drugs of abuse *alter mood*. These mood-altering drugs change brain chemicals and brain cells in a way that affects one's mood regardless of the circumstances. As a wise alcohol and drug counselor put it, "All these drugs do is fool your brain. You're still anxious or in pain." Mood-altering drugs allow a person to avoid facing reality temporarily. Unfortunately, those who attempt to avoid reality in the short term eventually end up colliding with it, usually in a painful way.

There is a major difference between mood-altering drugs and drugs that are used to treat conditions like depression or anxiety disorders. This point is frequently misunderstood, especially among recovering addicts and concerned family members. If you have clinical depression or panic disorder, the part of your brain that handles emotions is not functioning correctly, with resulting symptoms such as crying, irritability, nervousness, and sleeping problems. There are usually external factors causing you to be upset, and the brain is not handling those issues in the way it is supposed to. Medications that are prescribed for depression or anxiety disorders work within brain cells to prompt them to function properly. Most of these medications take time to get into the system and become effective. The benefit is not immediate. But a more important distinction is that these medications permit you to function optimally, so that you are better able to deal with reality. Your sense of being in control increases and your coping skills improve.

This is not so with mood-altering drugs. No matter what the condition of your brain at the time you start using, it will be changed. These drugs tend to override normal systems in the brain to produce an artificial mood state. When they leave your system, though, there is a rebound effect. The brain is going to resist this kind of unnatural override, and will not get back to normal for some time. To fight the effects of depressants, it becomes overactive; to fight the effect of stimulants, it becomes sluggish and depressed.

## Tolerance and Withdrawal

Tolerance is associated with various drugs and involves a number of different body systems; it is particularly noticeable where addictive substances are concerned. It is a phenomenon whereby the body develops an ability to tolerate the effects of a drug. This means that the body has made adjustments to overcome the drug's effects, which then causes the rebound effect referred to above.

With alcohol, there may also be a built-in tolerance in some people who have a family history of alcoholism. This accounts for the low response factor explained in the section on genetics.

Tolerance to alcohol and the depressants involves adaptive changes that up-regulate systems activating the central nervous system. In other words, the brain becomes hyperalert and hypersensitive in order to compensate. Tolerance to the opiates involves a similar process, although different pathways are in use.

Another type of tolerance involves the body's ability to metabolize the drug. Some drugs, such as the barbiturates, stimulate cells in the liver which break down and help eliminate drugs of all types. The rate of elimination of the drug goes up, so the amount needed to produce a clinical effect goes up as well. For this reason, people who are addicted to some types of drugs require higher than normal doses of other drugs to achieve an effect.

Cross-tolerance to similar substances is quite common. For example, if you develop tolerance to one type of depressant drug, you will have increased tolerance to other depressant drugs. Alcohol, barbiturates, and benzodiazepines are all cross-tolerant, so benzodiazepines such as Librium can be used to treat alcohol withdrawal and phenobarbital can be used to treat withdrawal from benzodiazepines. But this can also lead to cross-addiction. For example, an alcoholic might be inappropriately treated by a doctor's prescribing tranquilizers for "nerves" (really chronic withdrawal), which results in a cross-addiction. The person might not need to drink alcohol anymore, but the addiction is still there and active. Exposure to barbiturates or benzodiazepines can also trigger a relapse in a person who has been abstinent from alcohol, or vice versa.

One important system involved with alcohol and the depressants involves the overall electrical stability of the brain. Seizures, or convulsions, are episodes of unregulated electrical discharge within the brain. In order for a seizure to occur, one of two things has to happen. The first is that there has to be a strong stimulus. The second is that this stimulus has to override the regulatory mechanisms in each cell membrane. Seizures can be produced in two ways, by the addition of a strong electrical stimulus or by a decrease in the cell membranes' ability to resist the stimulus. When a person develops tolerance to alcohol or to the depressant medications, alterations in the function of a chemical that regulates the movement of calcium in and out of the cells causes these cells to be very sensitive to any kind of stimulation. The cells are unstable, so it takes little provocation to produce a seizure.

The withdrawal symptoms that we typically see in those who have used alcohol or the depressants expose the changes that the brain made when it developed tolerance to the effects of the substance. Shakiness, anxiety, irritability, and sometimes psychotic reactions are seen in people whose bodies are reacting to the absence of a depressant drug. Fatigue, sleepiness, depressed mood, and increased appetite are the symptoms in someone whose brain is reacting to the absence of stimulants.

Withdrawal symptoms emerge as the drug clears the system. With drugs that clear quickly, such as cocaine or alcohol, there is a fairly rapid onset of such symptoms. Other drugs clear very slowly, marijuana being the best example. This drug clears the body over the span of days to weeks. There has been much controversy over whether or not marijuana is physically addictive because of the lack of a distinct withdrawal syndrome. It has, however, been demonstrated that such a syndrome exists; it is simply hard to detect, because, as the drug slowly clears the system, the body gradually adapts. Nonetheless, it is probably just uncomfortable enough to make the resumption of use psychologically reinforcing.

It is also important to note that tolerance to drugs develops unevenly. Tolerance may develop to one effect of the drug and not to another. All drugs have a number of effects other than the desired ones. For example, tranquilizers such as the benzodiazepines (Valium and others) are useful for the short-term treatment of anxiety. However, they consistently cause drowsiness, and this is a "side effect" when the drug is prescribed for anxiety. Some drugs in this same class, though, are marketed for sleep. In this case the intended effect is the sedation. Tolerance to the sedative effects of these drugs will develop over time, which limits their long-term use as sleep aids. However, tolerance to the effect of relieving pathological anxiety does not develop to any substantial degree. Many people with severe anxiety disorders, therefore, are effectively maintained on these (and other) medications without a need to substantially increase the dose. Since tolerance to the drowsiness occurs over time, this side effect diminishes. So here is a situation where tolerance to one effect—sedation—is a problem in one type of case and an advantage in another.

However, development of tolerance to the desired effect of the drug can leave the person vulnerable to problems with other effects. For example, one of the effects of the opiates (such as heroin) is euphoria—an abnormal elevation of mood. Tolerance to this effect occurs rapidly, so that higher and higher doses are required to achieve the effect. Another effect of opiates is the depression of the respiratory reflex in the brain. Tolerance to this effect does not occur rapidly, if at all. As increasing doses of opiates are used, the person comes nearer and nearer to the toxic level. Death from an overdose of opiates is frequently due to the depression of the respiratory reflex.

Another example is cocaine, which also causes euphoria. Tolerance to this effect develops rapidly, leading the user to increase the dose or the frequency of use. Cocaine, however, also has what is known as a chronotropic effect on the heart, meaning that the drug speeds up the heart rate by stimulating that muscle to contract more rapidly. This can lead to heart damage. In fact, before the epidemic of cocaine dependence that reached its peak in the late 1980s, heart attacks in people under the age of thirty-five or forty were considered extremely rare. Then emergency rooms were suddenly seeing heart patients in their twenties, or even in their teens, because of the toxic effect of cocaine on the heart.

So the development of tolerance increases the dangerousness of the drug and also creates a situation in which the body becomes uncomfortable without it.

### Behavioral Conditioning and Craving

One of the fascinating things about addiction and the brain is that there is no single factor that causes addiction. As we have seen, it is not purely genetic, psychological, chemical, or behavioral. Every time you learn something, there is a chemical change in your brain that causes you to remember what you learned.

Some types of learning are conscious and intentional. Studying for a test is an example. This is called instrumental learning. An instrumental learning process that occurs when people begin to experiment with mood-altering drugs involves several tasks. The first is learning how to obtain access to the substance; then the user has to learn how to administer it and to manage its effect.

But there is another kind of learning that occurs at a more subliminal level. This is called conditioning, and it occurs when the brain learns to associate a particular effect with a certain situation.

The most familiar example of classical conditioning is the experiment involving Pavlov's dog. Pavlov was a Russian psychologist interested in the phenomenon of learning and memory. He rang a bell every time he fed his dog, and after a while found that the dog would salivate whenever the bell was rung, whether food was present or not. This important experiment showed that an animal's body "learned" to change its physiology based upon an environmental cue. (We cannot normally control functions like salivating, increased heart rate, sweating, or blushing, which occur in response to environmental stimuli.)

Experiments with addicts have shown that exposure to drug-related sensory cues produces changes in heart rate, pupil size, skin conductance, and the subjective feeling of craving. There is a direct correlation between the strength of these responses and the severity of the addiction.

Addicts in methadone treatment programs have reported

the onset of withdrawal symptoms in response to stressful emotions. When the methadone level in the bloodstream is constant, there is no biochemical reason for the addict to be in withdrawal. In this situation the brain has apparently "learned" that motivating the addict to use—by producing symptoms of withdrawal—will lead to the sense of relief that comes from a dose of opiates, even when they are already present in the system.

Cocaine addicts routinely report that they begin craving whenever they encounter sights, smells, and sounds that were common when and where they used cocaine. In fact, cocaine addicts in treatment centers often do not experience much in the way of craving, and may come to believe that this is not going to be a problem. However, when they return home, environmental cues trigger cravings.

In a number of treatment approaches, attempts have been made to take advantage of this effect or to reverse it. Aversive conditioning was tried for a short period of time, but is currently considered ineffective and probably unethical. In this treatment model, the addict is exposed to a stimulus that is likely to trigger craving, such as a bottle of alcohol or drug paraphernalia. When the automatic response occurs—pupil dilation, sweating, or subjective craving—a negative stimulus such as an electric shock is applied. The theory behind this approach is that the negative stimulus will become paired with the cue that triggers the craving, and therefore the strength of the addiction will be reduced. But the treatment didn't work very well and wasn't very popular.

Teaching addicts to deal with triggers and cravings, though, is an important part of current treatment approaches. Conditioned responses disappear over time. If, for example, Pavlov went for a long time without feeding the dog after the bell had been rung, the dog began to salivate less and less when it did ring.

We know that cravings peak in intensity and wane over a span of ten to fifteen minutes, providing that the addict does not use the drug and diverts his or her attention to something else. Drugs that are extremely addicting, like crack cocaine, produce the strongest conditioned responses and cravings. It can take a considerable period of time for these to diminish, but, if a person learns to avoid certain stimuli and stays completely abstinent, the cravings become more tolerable as they fade.

# 4. Alcohol and Addictive Drugs

The six large groups of mood-altering drugs are alcohol (beer, wine, distilled spirits), depressants (barbiturates, tranquilizers, sedatives, sleeping pills), stimulants (cocaine, amphetamines, caffeine, nicotine), opiates (heroin, opium, morphine, synthetic morphine compounds), hallucinogens (marijuana, LSD, PCP), and inhalants (nitrous oxide, toluene, gasoline).

## Alcohol

Alcohol has been around for centuries. It probably first appeared in skins full of grape juice that had been left out too long in the heat of the desert. Fruit syrup plus heat (and a few other ingredients) eventually produce ethanol, which is the active ingredient in all types of intoxicating beverages.

Alcohol is found in beer, wine, and distilled spirits. The active ingredient is the same—ethanol. The differences among these beverages is in the concentration of the alcohol. Beer is the most dilute, and the alcohol content varies from state to state. Wine is a little less dilute, and alcohol contents vary according to the type of wine. Less dilute are the distilled spirits, such as vodka or whiskey. Pure grain alcohol is the least dilute and is the substance known as "moonshine" or "corn squeezings."

Alcohol dissolves fat. The cells in our bodies are encased in membranes, which are complicated multilayered structures composed of specialized fats and proteins. They contain channels for various ions, such as calcium and potassium, and for messenger proteins that communicate with other cell structures which regulate the activity of the cell. Alcohol not only dissolves into the fats of the cell membrane but also disrupts many of these delicate structures.

But because it dissolves fat, alcohol crosses easily into all types of cells. This is one reason that drinking on an empty stomach makes a person drunk quickly. If there is nothing in the stomach, the alcohol crosses easily through the stomach lining and into the bloodstream, then through the blood-brain barrier, which is a specialized fatty membrane that protects the brain from many of the substances that get into the bloodstream. While it is exerting its intoxicating effects on the brain, it is also passing into the cells of various other organs in the body. This results in a variety of toxic effects.

What happens when you drink? In the short term, alcohol causes mild stimulation at first. It causes an easing of tension, a mild sense of euphoria, and a slight drop in inhibitions. It is for these effects that alcohol is used in social settings. But these occur only at low blood levels of alcohol.

As blood levels increase, the depressant effects become more obvious. Since alcohol affects the balance center of the brain, you become uncoordinated. Another part of the brain that becomes less functional is the frontal lobe area, which is the one that exercises social judgment. You might begin to make remarks that are inappropriate or do things that will seem embarrassing later. You might become irritable and easily provoked. Speech becomes slurred, and fine motor coordination is lost. Your ability to perform complex tasks such as driving is lost. And your ability to judge whether or not it's appropriate to drive is also lost.

As blood levels rise further, you may become stuporous and eventually lose consciousness. This is not quite the same as going to sleep, since it is a drug-induced state. The normal patterns of sleep, such as alternating periods of deep sleep and dreaming, are disrupted. At this point, the danger exists of an alcohol-induced coma with total depression of life functions such as the breathing reflex. Far too often we hear about teenagers or young adults who have intentionally drunk to a point of extreme intoxication and have ended up dead from respiratory arrest due to the alcohol.

Because the chemical structure of alcohol is fairly simple, one would expect it to have a number of diverse effects on the brain, and it does. Unlike some other addictive substances, alcohol does not interact directly with specific neurotransmitter systems. But it does interfere with the activity of a number of substances important in the regulation of mood and excitability of the brain. Alcohol also has a cascading effect on several systems in the brain, probably produced in part by the effects that it has on the fats within the membranes of nerve cells. Each of these intoxicating effects reflects alcohol's interaction with and disruption of a different brain system. We can break down the intoxicating effect of alcohol on the brain into four basic categories: mood-altering effects, motor impairment, interference with memory, reasoning, and judgment, and addictive potential.

The research literature on the molecular effects of alcohol is very complicated, so we'll just touch the high points. Alcohol has been found to cause short-term and long-term changes in a number of chemical systems, including those of the neurotransmitters GABA (gamma amino butyric acid), norepinephrine, serotonin, dopamine, adenosine, and choline. Changes in these systems are felt to account for most of alcohol's intoxicating effects.

The addictive potential of alcohol arises from two sources. As the brain adapts to the substance's widespread intoxicating effects, it adjusts its internal regulating systems to compensate. So when you stop drinking, you experience some very unpleasant sensations, including anxiety, depression, shakiness, inability to sleep, and irritability. Drinking alcohol again brings the system back into equilibrium—for a while. It is reinforcing, then, to drink again, and the cycle continues. It was initially thought that this was the basis of addiction to alcohol—drinking to avoid the effects of withdrawal. But it goes further than that.

As we have learned, addicting drugs interact at some point within the ventral tegmentum or medial forebrain bundle, structures that make up the pleasure center of the brain. Several lines of evidence suggest that alcohol has an effect, probably indirectly, on the dopamine system in this part of the brain. Research indicates that there may be genetic differences in the sensitivity of the dopamine system to alcohol. Evidence also exists that alcohol affects the opiate system of the brain. The suggestion is that there may be genetic differences in play here, too.

The research so far supports the long-standing observation that there appear to be different types of alcoholics. Some alcoholics seem to be as highly addicted to alcohol as heroin or crack addicts are to their drugs of choice. Others have less craving when dry, but lose control of the amount they drink. Genetic differences in how the brain responds to the effects of alcohol might explain this difference.

Longer-term effects of alcohol fall into two categories: adaptive changes in the brain and direct toxicity. As we saw in the section on tolerance, the brain adapts to the presence of a mood-altering drug by trying to bring the system back into equilibrium. With alcohol, the overall effect is to crank up the brain's alerting system so that a person can have more alcohol in his or her system without experiencing the depressant effects. Over the long term, this leads to a situation that we call chronic withdrawal, which means that the whole central nervous system remains hyperactive even if the person is drinking on a regular basis. It is even possible for someone with severe alcoholism to begin to have the symptoms of DTs (delirium tremens) with alcohol still in the system. Alcoholics commonly have generalized seizures while drinking heavily due to this hyperactivity and oversensitivity of the central nervous system.

Other symptoms of chronic withdrawal (or the long-term adaptation of the brain to the presence of alcohol) can be both physical and psychological. High blood pressure is a common physical manifestation, as are chronic sinus congestion and a low-grade tremor. People dependent on alcohol also complain of a variety of psychological symptoms including irritability, anxiety, panic attacks, depression, mood swings, and paranoia. These symptoms reflect the long-term adaptation of the brain to the presence of alcohol and eventually clear with abstinence. Most symptoms are markedly better within two weeks of detoxification, although some emotional instability may remain for several months.

Although alcohol is legally produced, sold, and used in our society, it is one of the most toxic substances on our list of addictive drugs. It is toxic to several organ systems in the body, including the liver, bone marrow, brain, heart, stomach lining, and pancreas.

When alcohol is metabolized in the liver, it causes a general inflammation, which leads to the development of fatty deposits in liver cells. Over time, with repeated inflammation due to alcohol, some people develop scarring in the liver, which leads to cirrhosis. The word "cirrhosis" literally means "scarring." As these scars form between liver cells, the liver contracts and becomes hardened, resulting in a reduced ability of the liver to perform its function of clearing wastes from the system. It also blocks the flow of blood through the liver. Blood in the large veins coming out of the abdomen starts to back up, resembling a clogged drainage system. This results in symptoms such as hemorrhoids or fluid collection in the abdomen. Over the long term, bulging areas occur in large veins in such places as the esophagus, and these can rupture, leading to serious hemorrhage. The liver also produces important clotting factors, and a damaged liver leads to problems with slow blood clotting. A hemorrhage in this situation is very serious. Since the liver is not clearing wastes, a build-up of ammonia can occur in the blood-stream, leading to inflammation of the brain and decreased consciousness.

Alcohol is toxic to the bone marrow as well. The cells that are the forerunners of mature blood cells are damaged, and larger, less mature red blood cells are released into the system. Alcohol also damages the immune system, with the result that alcoholics are more prone to a variety of serious infections.

Alcohol has several specific toxic effects on the brain. Many alcoholics become deficient in vitamin B-1, or thiamine. A part of the brain that is important in the processing and storing of memory is particularly sensitive to the combined effect of the vitamin deficiency and the presence of alcohol. When this part of the brain is destroyed, it causes the person to lose the capacity to retain any new information. Alcohol also is destructive to the cerebellum, the part of the brain that controls balance and muscle movement. In some individuals, the part of the brain that connects the two hemispheres is also damaged, and there seems to be a hereditary disposition to this type of brain damage. Some alcoholics develop auditory hallucinations, which are voices that are usually derisive and unpleasant. This also seems to be due to brain damage caused by the alcohol. And, in addition, alcohol causes generalized damage to all nerve cells, which can lead to dementia, or loss of intellectual functioning. This can be quite severe, rendering the person in need of supervised institutional care.

Alcohol damages muscle tissue, which is most serious when the damage occurs to the heart muscle. Alcoholic cardiomyopathy is a condition in which the heart muscle has been damaged, and is flabby and dilated. When the heart does not pump effectively, heart failure results. Also, the heart beats in an uncoordinated fashion, compounding the problem.

Alcohol is toxic as well to the lining of the stomach and the digestive tract. It is not uncommon for people to have

acute gastritis (irritation of the stomach) following a drinking
binge. This can cause pinpoint bleeding, which results in
vomiting, diarrhea, and anemia. If this happens in a person
with cirrhosis, it can result in a disastrous gastrointestinal
hemorrhage.

Alcohol irritates the pancreas, an organ lying beneath
the stomach across from the liver. Its function is to produce
digestive enzymes and insulin. When it is inflamed, it releases
its digestive enzymes and begins to destroy itself. This is a
very painful condition. Furthermore, repeated episodes of
pancreatic inflammation eventually damage the cells that make
insulin. Without insulin, the body cannot control blood sugar,
and this causes a diabetic condition.

Alcohol, which is socially acceptable and legal in most
countries, is one of the most toxic of the addictive drugs to
all body systems. Even social drinkers, who do not develop
addiction to alcohol, are not immune to its toxicity.

### Depressants

The depressants include several classes of pharmaceutical
drugs, mainly developed and marketed as sleep aids, tranquilizers, anesthetic agents, muscle relaxers, and anticonvulsants.
Inappropriate prescribing and illegal diversion are the two
main sources of these drugs on the street, although some "pi-
rated" versions imported from illegal labs are also available.

The two most common varieties of depressants we encounter are the barbiturates, such as Seconal and Tuinal, and
the benzodiazepines, such as Valium and Xanax. Other less
common and older depressants include such compounds as
Quaalude (no longer legally available in the United States),
chloral hydrate (the active ingredient in a Mickey Finn),
paraldehyde (widely used in the past to treat severe alcohol
withdrawal), and obsolete tranquilizers such as Placidyl,
Miltown, and Equanil.

## Barbiturates

The barbiturates have been around for quite a while, and are used primarily as general anesthetics and anticonvulsants. In the past they were used as tranquilizers and sleeping pills, but this practice has diminished, for safety reasons, since the benzodiazepines became available.

The barbiturates act in a dose-related fashion. At low doses they produce mild sedation. With increasing doses, this effect progresses from sleep to anesthesia to respiratory depression to death. These drugs also have a low therapeutic index, meaning that the dose required for the desired effect— sedation, sleep or anesthesia—is very close to the toxic dose.

People suffering from barbiturate overdose, an extremely dangerous situation, were once commonly seen in emergency rooms. Often these overdoses were accidental. The user, having begun to develop tolerance to the drug's sedative effects, would repeat the dose. (This was alleged to have been the cause of Marilyn Monroe's death.)

Barbiturates cause addiction in two ways. A person can develop a physical dependence on the effects of the barbiturate as tolerance develops to the sedative effects. Stopping these drugs abruptly will lead to symptoms of withdrawal. Withdrawal from barbiturates is very dangerous, involving agitation, anxiety, muscle cramps, seizures, delirium, and possibly death. Repetitive use of barbiturates to avoid the symptoms of withdrawal contributes to the addiction. But barbiturates also interact with the pleasure center of the brain to produce the same reinforcing response caused by other drugs of addiction.

## Benzodiazepines

The benzodiazepines include drugs such as Valium, Xanax, Restoril, Dalmane, and Ativan. At one point they were among the most commonly prescribed drugs in the nation. They are remarkably safe from a medical standpoint—they do not cause much in the way of toxic side effects, and they are not nearly as lethal as barbiturates in the case of an overdose. They are effective for the short-term treatment of anxiety and insomnia. For psychiatric disorders such as panic disorder, they can be used under medical supervision for long periods of time without losing effectiveness.

But they are mood altering, and they have addictive potential. These drugs interact with receptors for the neurotransmitter GABA (gamma amino butyric acid). When GABA is activated, it has a calming effect on the central nervous system, closely related to the brain's pleasure center, so these drugs have a reinforcing ability similar to that of the barbiturates, but are less potent.

The addictive potential of benzodiazepines is relatively low compared to the barbiturates or to drugs like heroin or cocaine. It is unusual to find a person with addiction whose main drug of choice is a benzodiazepine. Street use of these drugs is usually in combination with other drugs. For example, alcoholics use them to treat hangovers and symptoms of chronic withdrawal; cocaine and amphetamine addicts do so to soften the effects of the "crash" or to modulate the high of the stimulant effect. However, there are cases in which people abuse prescriptions for benzodiazepines. Such individuals are generally relying on the drug's effects to help them cope with stress, and they tend to increase the prescribed dose or to run out of their prescriptions early. These people often have past problems with substance abuse or have a family history of addiction.

It's important to mention at this point that the mere fact that a person has a physiological dependence on these medications does not mean that there is an addiction present. For example, many people with anxiety disorders have been maintained successfully for many years on medications like Ativan or Xanax. There are also people with seizure disorders that are managed with phenobarbital. If they were to stop taking these medications abruptly, they would experience withdrawal symptoms. So whenever these drugs are stopped after more than several months of use, a slow tapering off should be done under medical supervision. A physiological dependence is not in itself a reason to stop the drug if it is being used properly under medical supervision.

Withdrawal from depressant medications is serious business and usually requires hospitalization for detoxification. Symptoms can include agitation, insomnia, seizures, hallucinations, and confusion. Withdrawal symptoms from some of the benzodiazepines don't occur immediately, since these drugs take a while to clear out of the system. So it's not uncommon for extreme discomfort to develop many days after the last dose. And some mild symptoms, like insomnia and uneasiness, can persist for several months. People getting through the first three or four months without benzodiazepines can find it pretty tough going, and I generally approach these patients with a great deal of patience and encouragement, assuring them that if they can just wait, it will get better.

### Stimulants

Stimulant drugs, or "uppers," include cocaine and the amphetamines. Substances such as ephedrine, pseudoephedrine, and phenylpropanoloamine are also classified as stimulants. These drugs are available as over-the-counter decongestants, diet aids, and stimulants. Caffeine, found in coffee, tea, colas, cocoa, and over-the-counter drugs, is also a stimulant. Nicotine is included in this section since it has some stimulant properties and closely resembles the stimulants with respect to withdrawal symptoms and associated cravings.

All of the stimulants act in one way or another to increase the activity of a part of the central nervous system known as the sympathetic nervous system, which is what causes us to be on alert and produces the fight or flight reaction. It functions in a balanced fashion with the parasympathetic nervous system, which controls functions such as eating, digesting, and slowing the heart rate. Norepinephrine, which is closely related to adrenaline, is the main neurotransmitter involved in the activity of the sympathetic nervous system.

When your sympathetic nervous system is active, several things occur. Blood vessels in the gut constrict, leading to a reduced appetite. Blood flow to the brain and muscles increases. Your heart rate goes up, as does your blood pressure. Pupils dilate, and in extreme cases your hair stands on end. Your senses become more acute, and you are more alert. Your ability to concentrate goes up. To a mild degree, these effects are pleasurable to most people.

Caffeine, nicotine, and over-the-counter preparations produce these effects to a mild degree if they're used in moderation. Cocaine and amphetamines are much more potent, and have much more potential for abuse. The use of intravenous or smoked forms of stimulants leads to an intense and highly addictive sensation and also to the development of cravings when the drug is stopped.

Stimulant addicts typically use in an episodic fashion. The user will binge for several days (periods called runs) and then crash. During the crash, the user will experience depression, fatigue, agitation, and craving. Cocaine or amphetamine addicts will often abuse depressant drugs, opiates, or alcohol during the crash to modulate the symptoms.

### Cocaine

Cocaine is found naturally in the leaves of the coca plant, which grows in high altitude areas of South America. The ancient Incas chewed these leaves for their mild stimulant effect, which resembles that of a strong cup of coffee. The practice is still in effect. The amount of drug that is delivered in this fashion is rather low, and it does not pose a major health problem. But distilling the active ingredient—cocaine—from the coca plant produces a much more potent substance. Processed cocaine has been used for at least a century, for a variety of purposes.

When applied to tissue, cocaine produces local anesthesia. A legitimate use of cocaine is found in the operating room. Cocaine spray is applied before the insertion of breathing tubes used during surgery. Cocaine's stimulant effects have also been long recognized. Sigmund Freud had advocated the use of cocaine for a variety of medical indications before coming to understand the drug's addictive potential and retracting any such recommendations.

Cocaine acts directly on brain cells within the pleasure center by stimulating the release of dopamine and other neurotransmitters. It essentially overrides the natural control mechanisms of this system, which leads to the intensely pleasurable high but also to an eventual depletion of the stores of these chemicals. Cocaine users eventually lose the ability to feel this pleasurable sensation as the stores are depleted further and further and the brain becomes tolerant to the drug's effects.

But the drug also sets up a strong conditioning effect leading to severe cravings. Within a short period of time, the user is caught between the strength of the cravings and the dull depression that results when the drug is not present in the system. It can take many months for the brain to build the stores of neurotransmitters back up. Irritability, severe depression, hallucinations, and delusions can result from the chronic use of cocaine. Sudden mood swings and episodes of uncharacteristic hostility and abusiveness may be observed by family members and coworkers who may be unaware of the addiction.

Cocaine is abused in several forms. Powder cocaine is inhaled nasally. The substance can be altered chemically through a process of free-basing and administered intravenously or by inhalation. Crack or rock cocaine is formed from powder cocaine, and comes in small crystals that resemble chunks of soap. These are burned in a pipe or another vehicle and inhaled. One crack rock can be relatively inexpensive, making them widely accessible, but it's not uncommon for a crack addict to spend as much money as is available—and more—to repeat the brief high over and over again.

It has been something of a rule of thumb that most addicts have a particular drug of choice, or a category of choice. For example, people who do "downers" generally don't like the effects of stimulants and vice versa. However, crack cocaine has proven to be the great leveler in this regard—when crack cocaine is available, many addicts of all types eventually end up using it primarily, while occasionally drinking or using other drugs such as the depressants to deal with side effects.

### Amphetamines

The amphetamines include legitimate pharmaceutical preparations as well as illicitly produced substances. Amphetamines have been used medically as bronchodilators for asthma, appetite depressants for weight loss, in treatment of attention deficit disorder in children and of narcolepsy, and as a supplement in the treatment of some forms of resistant depression. During World War II and the Vietnam war, amphetamines were made available to troops to help counteract fatigue and improve concentration.

During the 1960s and 1970s, the illicit use of amphetamines became widespread. A large proportion of the drugs came from the diversion of legitimately produced pharmaceutical preparations. As a result of increased regulatory efforts, it is less common now to find drugs such as Dexedrine or Benzedrine on the streets. Instead, the supply of crystal methamphetamine produced in illegal labs has grown. "Cooking" crystal meth is relatively easy and quite lucrative, although it is extremely dangerous. The chemicals used to create the drug are toxic and highly explosive. Crystal meth addiction tends to cluster in certain parts of the country, such as the South and the Southwest, close to the illicit labs. It's also frequently abused by long-haul truckers. In some cases, crack cocaine addicts have turned to crystal meth as a substitute because of the lower cost and longer high.

Amphetamines exert their effect on the brain in a twofold fashion. They attach to and directly stimulate the cells that produce excitation of certain areas of the brain. They also cause these cells to secrete neurotransmitters like norepinephrine and dopamine, which also contribute to the stimulating and euphoric effects. The main problem with the amphetamines is that, in overriding the brain's normal regulatory mechanisms, they cause profound depletion of the brain's normal chemicals, just as cocaine does. Even months after cessation of use, lab animals demonstrate lower than normal levels of important neurotransmitters like norepinephrine, dopamine, and serotonin. It is thought that in some cases of long-term, heavy use, these chemicals never return to normal levels.

Long-term, heavy use of amphetamines leads to a psychosis that is clinically indistinguishable from paranoid schizophrenia. "Speed freaks" become intensely paranoid, and may experience hallucinations. Amphetamines also trigger seriously aggressive behavior, especially if the user feels threatened. Physical effects of the stimulant properties of amphetamines can lead to major physical complications such as heart damage, strokes, and life-threatening fevers.

Amphetamines are similar to other stimulant drugs in how they produce addiction. There is a powerful conditioning effect. The brain learns to associate a pleasurable sensation with all kinds of cues connected to the use of the drug. During the early period of abstinence, as with cocaine, the addict has to deal with powerful cravings that are a result of this learning process.

### Caffeine

Caffeine is probably the most widely used mood-altering substance. It is found in coffee, tea, cola, cocoa, and over-the-counter analgesics and stimulants. It's not associated with any kind of social or serious health problem and is therefore not considered dangerous enough to regulate. It does, however, have some troublesome effects that are worth knowing about.

The term "caffeinism" refers to a group of symptoms caused by excessive, chronic ingestion of the substance, including restlessness, nervousness, and muscle twitching, as well as some gastrointestinal problems. It's a common cause of insomnia or restless sleep. For people with depression or anxiety disorders, caffeine can aggravate symptoms and complicate treatment.

Withdrawal symptoms begin to emerge and peak within a day or two after the last ingestion of caffeine. These symptoms can include fatigue, headache, irritability, withdrawal, and poor concentration. It's not uncommon for people who drink coffee all day long during the work week to experience caffeine withdrawal on the weekends or during vacations. The easiest way to diagnose caffeine withdrawal is to have the sufferer drink a cup of coffee or a Coke and see what happens. Weekend headache sufferers who get relief from over-the-counter preparations that contain caffeine are unwittingly treating the withdrawal.

### Nicotine

Addiction to nicotine is probably the most prevalent drug problem in today's world. Nicotine is found in tobacco products such as cigarettes, cigars, pipe tobacco, chewing tobacco, and snuff. The addictiveness of nicotine is well documented, as are the health hazards of smoking and chewing tobacco.

Nicotine acts as a stimulant in a fashion similar to that of cocaine and amphetamines; however, its overall effect is less pronounced. It also interacts with a number of other systems in the brain such as the cholinergic system and hormonal systems. It has reinforcing properties caused by its interaction with dopamine-producing cells in the pleasure center of the brain.

Smokers have been shown to unconsciously regulate their doses of nicotine to amazingly consistent levels. Even smokers who switch to "light" cigarettes eventually increase the number of cigarettes smoked or the depth of inhalation to keep the nicotine levels constant.

Nicotine's effects are immediate and short-lived. Smokers generally begin to crave another cigarette within a few hours of the last one, and it is thought that the primary mechanism for addiction to cigarettes is that of treating the symptoms of withdrawal. In other words, the immediate reduction of anxiety and irritability that comes from smoking another cigarette tends to reinforce the addiction.

Although nicotine addiction does not cause the profound social and behavioral problems that result from the use of drugs like cocaine and amphetamines, it is associated with many serious medical problems, including cancer and heart disease. Quitting smoking is no easy matter, and there are high failure rates for all methods. Nonetheless, social pressure has encouraged many people to be successful in their efforts. It may be that as smoking becomes more and more socially unacceptable, the remaining smokers will be people with more complicated problems. For example, smoking is more prevalent among people who are addicted to other substances and among those with other psychiatric problems. The reasons for this are not completely clear, but it's probably because the brain is so complicated and nicotine's effects are fairly widespread throughout the nervous system. Changing the system by eliminating nicotine may cause a cascade of effects in people whose brains are otherwise abnormal, which would make quitting much more complicated.

## Over-the-Counter Stimulants

A number of fairly powerful stimulants are available on the shelves of the drugstore and health food store. Among these are ephedrine and pseudoephedrine preparations and the compound phenylpropanolamine, which is commonly found in over-the-counter diet aids. These preparations are relatively safe if used as directed, but are often misused. Ephedrine and related compounds closely resemble amphetamines in chemical structure. Recent research has confirmed the ability of ephedrine to produce the same lever-pushing behavior that is seen in lab animals exposed to other addictive drugs.

Primary addictions to over-the-counter stimulants are uncommon but may be more prevalent than we know, since these drugs are not regulated and often doctors do not ask about them when taking medical histories. It is important that people who are recovering from addictions know that these compounds may trigger relapse or cause a problem with cross-addiction.

## Opiates

The opiates are derived from a naturally occurring substance, morphine, which comes from a specific variety of the poppy plant. There are naturally occurring opiates such as morphine and heroin and synthetically produced ones such as meperidine (Demerol) and propoxyphene (Darvon). As we've learned, there are also opiate-like substances called endorphins that are produced naturally in the brain.

Opiates have a number of diverse actions in the body. In addition to pain relief, they provide a sense of euphoria and relaxation. This effect may be more pronounced in people who are addicted or who are at risk genetically for addiction. There are also people who feel uncomfortable and uneasy when using opiates for pain relief. This constitutional difference is intriguing, and probably reflects differences in the genetic vulnerability to addiction to these drugs.

Opiates suppress the cough reflex and therefore are found in many cough preparations. They decrease the motility of the gastrointestinal tract and have a pharmaceutical use as a treatment for diarrhea. Opiates also cause the pupils to become constricted, provoke nausea, and are involved in the regulation of body temperature.

The pain-relieving effects of opiates have been appreciated for thousands of years; addiction to them has most likely been a problem for at least as long. When the brain is exposed to opiates such as morphine, physical tolerance and dependence develop, even at very low doses. It has been shown, for example, that hospital patients who are given even small doses of opiate medications for acute pain have a "mini" withdrawal syndrome even after the first dose. This does not mean that the patient has an addiction to opiates. It does mean that the brain reacts very quickly and strongly to the potentially addictive effects of these drugs. And, as with the benzodiazepines, a person can have a physiological dependence on an opiate drug because of medical use without becoming an addict. This is because there is more to addiction that just the body's reaction to the drug; behavioral, psychological, and spiritual factors play a role as well. Supervised medical detoxification from long-term use of opiate analgesics for acutely painful conditions such as burns will correct any physiological dependence. Continuing someone on opiate analgesics when physiological dependence exists is appropriate if the pain cannot be managed in any other way, as, for example, with cancer.

I generally see two types of opiate addiction. The first is heroin addiction, which was widespread in the sixties and seventies, dropped off during the crack cocaine epidemic in the eighties, and is coming back at the turn of the century. Heroin is a simple derivative of morphine which is not active when taken orally. In the past, it was typically injected

intravenously (mainlined). We are now seeing people addicted
to smoking or snorting heroin. They are able to avoid the risk
of AIDS associated with dirty needles, but the addiction to
the heroin is no less severe.

The second type is addiction to pharmaceutical opiate
preparations. These include drugs such as meperidine (Demerol), pentazocine (Talwin), propoxyphene (Darvocet), and
hydrocodone (Lorcet). This type of addiction usually starts
when there is easy access to these medications and then
progresses. Medical personnel, such as doctors and nurses,
often become addicted to these drugs. People with chronic
pain or headaches may begin to self-medicate emotional
pain with prescription opiates. When addiction develops,
these people frequently exaggerate their pain complaints,
feign painful conditions such as kidney stones or migraines,
and maintain multiple prescriptions from different doctors
at various pharmacies. It can sometimes be difficult to tell
the difference between someone with legitimate complaints
of chronic pain and someone who uses these complaints to
further an addiction, but careful evaluation and follow-up
usually make it possible to handle a situation appropriately.

Several types of opiate receptors have different functions in
the brain. Designing synthetic drugs that target only specific
receptors may lead to effective pain medications that are less
likely to cause addiction. One of these drugs is tramadol
(Ultram), which is said to provide good pain relief without
addiction potential. However, there are reports of people
abusing or appearing to become dependent on tramadol, so
the verdict is not yet in. It should be noted that meperidine
(Demerol) was first thought to have this quality, but it turned
out to be highly addictive. Tramadol should probably be
used with caution until there is more experience with this
drug, especially for people with a history of addiction. An
intriguing development is the finding that tramadol may
provide useful treatment for some psychiatric disorders, such
as obsessive-compulsive disorder. It will be interesting to

follow developments in the area of the opiate receptors and their differing functions.

The withdrawal syndrome associated with opiate addiction reflects the diverse actions of the opiates in the body. The term "cold turkey" was coined to describe what the withdrawing heroin addict looks like—shivering and covered with goose flesh.

The onset of withdrawal symptoms depends on how long it takes the drug or drugs to leave the system. Half-life is the measurement of the time it takes for one half of a drug to leave. Opiates with a short half-life, such as meperidine (Demerol) or heroin, leave the system within a matter of hours, and the onset of withdrawal symptoms follows soon after. Methadone, on the other hand, has a very long half-life, around one or two days.

Symptoms of opiate withdrawal include craving, muscle cramps, diarrhea, yawning, sweating, and runny nose, elevated temperature, and poor sleep. The condition has been compared to a case of the flu. Opiate withdrawal, unlike withdrawal from alcohol or the depressants, is more uncomfortable than it is medically dangerous.

Withdrawal can be treated by replacing the short half-life drug, such as heroin, with a longer half-life drug, such as methadone, and gradually tapering it off. It can also be treated symptomatically with drugs such as clonidine that block the specific symptoms of withdrawal. The acute symptoms, if not treated, last about a week for drugs with a short half-life and about two weeks for methadone. A protracted withdrawal syndrome that is often seen after the initial detoxification from opiates may last for months. It involves chronic, low-grade depression and a lack of stress tolerance, sometimes accompanied by drug cravings. It's unclear whether this is a direct effect of the opiates or involves coexisting psychiatric problems.

The problem with treating opiate addiction has always been that there is a very high relapse rate. This may be due to the protracted withdrawal syndrome. One solution that is controversial is the use of methadone replacement for long-term treatment. A person in a methadone maintenance program remains physiologically dependent on opiates and participates in group and individual therapy to address the other aspects of the addiction. Since methadone has a long half-life, it can be administered under medical supervision at a clinic. The addict does not have to devote time and energy to locating and procuring the drug. Some people believe that abstinence is the only ideal road to recovery, but experience has shown that the quality of life of the street addict successfully maintained in a methadone program improves greatly. People are able to hold down jobs, take care of family responsibilities, and lead otherwise normal lives. There is a new drug with an even longer half-life called LAAM which may make maintenance programs more efficient since it needs to be given only weekly.

Opiates are not very toxic compared to other addictive substances like alcohol. The most common medical problem we see is overdose. This often happens when tolerance has developed to the mood-altering effects but not to the respiratory effects. The addict pushes the dose up to achieve a high, and respiratory arrest occurs accidentally. Obviously, street preparations of heroin are not standardized, and an unusually pure supply of heroin in the drug community often leads to an epidemic of overdose deaths.

Even though opiates themselves are relatively safe, opiate addicts are generally not well. The use of dirty needles leads to infections of all kinds, including AIDS. Drug supplies are "cut" with various substances, and these can cause serious organ damage when injected or smoked. Poor nutrition and poor hygiene also contribute to the development of infectious diseases. Pregnant addicts have many more complications with their pregnancies, and the infants are at risk for a variety of medical problems. There is some evidence that long-term exposure to opiates may permanently damage the endogenous opiate system of the addict's brain, leading to chronic depression and anxiety.

## Hallucinogens

The hallucinogens consist of natural and synthetic substances that alter perception. Peyote, a natural substance derived from cactus plants, is used in religious rituals by Native Americans in the Southwest. Hallucinogenic properties are found in several other natural substances including some fungi, mushrooms, and seeds. Ergot alkaloids, commonly found in moldy rye bread, have hallucinogenic properties, and may have accounted for the bizarre behaviors of the women involved in the Salem witch trials.

### Marijuana

Like the opiates, cocaine, and alcohol, marijuana has been around for thousands of years. The first recorded description of the intoxicating effects of marijuana is found in ancient Chinese accounts of its medical use, more than four thousand years ago.

The active ingredients of marijuana are found in the resins of the hemp plant, *Cannabis sativa*. This leafy plant grows wild in most warm climates and was cultivated in colonial America to make ropes and fishing nets from the fibrous portion of the stems. The leaves of the marijuana plant can be dried and smoked for an intoxicating effect, and the resin can be extracted and concentrated into other forms such as hash oil.

The question of whether marijuana is dangerous as an addictive drug is highly controversial and politicized. Marijuana was listed in the U.S. Pharmacopoeia as late as the 1940s as a remedy for cough, migraines, menstrual cramps, and other conditions. Extracts of the active marijuana resin were available as over-the-counter tonics in the nineteenth and early twentieth centuries.

In 1937 the Marihuana Tax Act [*sic*] was enacted at the federal level. Most states had already passed laws regulating the sale and use of marijuana. This was the era of alcohol prohibition, and the recreational use of marijuana had come to replace alcohol in some social circles. A propaganda campaign was launched, designed to heighten public fears about marijuana. By the late fifties and early sixties, this had backfired.

Marijuana had been touted to cause insanity, violence, debauchery, and other evils. Recreational users, on the other hand, experienced mild intoxication with very few adverse effects. Marijuana came to be widely used on college campuses and by those in the hippie movement, and eventually spread to other levels of society. Laws were passed to decriminalize the possession and use of marijuana, but it remains classified by the Drug Enforcement Administration as a Schedule I drug, along with drugs such as heroin and LSD, which are felt to be dangerous and without legitimate medical use. Stiff penalties remain in effect for the manufacture and sale of marijuana.

In the eighties and nineties, the use of marijuana for certain medical conditions began to attract widespread interest. Marijuana is known to reduce the pressure in the eye that causes glaucoma. It also stimulates appetite and helps counteract the violent nausea associated with cancer chemotherapy. It has been used in pain management and as a muscle relaxer or tranquilizer. Researchers have studied it extensively and have developed some pharmaceutical preparations, such as Marinol, which is used for its antinausea and appetite-stimulating properties. Making marijuana readily available for medical use remains highly controversial and problematic.

Our familiarity with what marijuana actually does in the brain is fairly limited compared with how much we know about other drugs like opiates or alcohol. Part of the problem lies in the fact that natural cannabis contains many different compounds, most of which are active in one way or another. It is generally agreed that the major active component of marijuana is a chemical known as delta-9 tetrahydrocannabinol, or THC. Those who use natural marijuana for various medical reasons contend, however, that THC alone does not have the same beneficial effect as the natural substance.

The effects of marijuana include general relaxation, a heightening of the senses, distortion of time sense, and mild euphoria. At high doses, it can cause hallucinations, paranoia, and anxiety. Physical effects include an increase in heart rate, dry mouth, impaired coordination, and delayed reaction time.

Controversy continues as to the drug's addictiveness. It was once thought that marijuana was not physically addicting because there was no observable withdrawal syndrome. But over the last several decades, improvements in the cultivation of marijuana have led to a marked increase in its potency. A withdrawal syndrome involving anxiety, insomnia, and tremors has since been described. But an important factor compounding the study of withdrawal symptoms is that marijuana has a very long half-life. As a result it tapers off slowly after use is terminated. Slow tapering is the method of detoxification from other drugs, and it would therefore make sense that a clinically significant withdrawal syndrome is not readily seen.

Marijuana has been shown to interact with the ventral tegmental area of the brain, as have other addictive drugs, and is likely to have the same reinforcing qualities. This interaction probably also accounts for the drug's mood-altering and euphoric effects. Marijuana is often used in combination with other addictive drugs such as alcohol and cocaine. Polysubstance dependence is the addiction to two or more substances. It is very common and often includes marijuana dependence. The possibility that marijuana use promotes addiction to other substances has not been well studied but might account for the fact that many addicts start out experimenting with nicotine, alcohol, or marijuana, and then later develop addiction to cocaine or opiates.

The long-term effects of marijuana also remain controversial. A syndrome of poor motivation and apathy (the amotivational syndrome) has been described in chronic marijuana users by some researchers and refuted by others. Marijuana's ability to produce or to trigger long-term psychiatric problems like schizophrenia has also been described by some and refuted by others.

So what is the truth about marijuana? I think it's best to look at the studies with a bit of skepticism and instead see what we can observe in people who get into trouble with drugs and alcohol. Although marijuana does not produce the intense craving that drugs like crack cocaine and heroin do, it does alter mood, which allows the user to avoid dealing with reality. And the more one avoids dealing with reality, the more problems one is going to have in life. Even people who use marijuana for medical reasons experience this alteration in mood; it does have a profound effect.

People recovering from dependence on marijuana often have to deal with the regret of missed opportunities, lost productivity, and ruined relationships. Marijuana impairs driving ability and causes accidents. It is a "gateway" drug, especially for young people, opening the door to experimentation with other drugs and exposing the user to the drug culture. Smoking marijuana causes lung damage at a much faster rate than smoking cigarettes does. Proponents of the legalization of marijuana ignore these dangers, or compare them to the dangers of alcohol, which is legal.

A few benign experiences with marijuana give the user a false sense of security because of the lack of immediate consequences. First-time users often feel, then, that everything they have heard about marijuana is a lie, so the warnings about other drugs must be a lie, too.

The bottom line is that marijuana is alive and well in the drug culture, and its use is well represented among people who seek treatment for drug dependence. Controlled medical use may be of benefit to some people, but, contrary to the assertions of those who push for full legalization of marijuana, it is not a benign natural herb. If you put the statistical studies down and just talk to people who are successfully recovering from addiction to marijuana, you will probably find that they take it very seriously.

### LSD, PCP, and Other Hallucinogens

In the early 1940s, a researcher working for the Sandoz pharmaceutical company stumbled upon the mind-altering qualities of LSD following an accidental ingestion. Sandoz has marketed a number of ergot derivatives, which have long had a place in medical use because they are effective in aborting migraine headaches. But this new compound had surprisingly profound effects unlike those seen with the migraine drugs. Scientists began to study the effects of the drug, looking for a potential application in medicine.

Psychiatrists studied the drug's potential use as a chemical that could enhance exploratory types of psychotherapy. At that time, treatment in psychiatry was based on the theory that psychoanalytic exploration of the unconscious would lead to the resolution of buried conflicts, which would result in the relief of symptoms. If a compound such as LSD could facilitate this process by loosening repression and bringing unconscious material to the fore, then it might be very useful.

LSD was used experimentally over the next two decades in a number of medical and military settings with some encouraging positive results, but there were also reports of serious adverse reactions such as suicides and psychosis. The eventual conclusion about LSD as a psychiatric drug was that, while interesting in its effects, it was not terribly useful and was potentially dangerous.

The rise in the popularity and street use of LSD was a phenomenon that reflected the cultural changes of the 1960s.

Dr. Timothy Leary, once an instructor at Harvard, was instrumental in popularizing the drug, and coined the term "psychedelic." Marijuana and LSD became popular symbols of the antiestablishment movement. The more the government objected to and preached against these drugs, the more popular they became. LSD lost much of its attractiveness after publicity about "bad trips" and about people doing dangerous things while under its influence, such as leaping from rooftops to their death because they thought they could fly. The use of LSD waned through the seventies and eighties, as the use of the combined hallucinogen/stimulant known as Ecstasy increased, but in the late nineties LSD made a comeback among teenagers and young adults.

Originally developed in the 1950s, PCP, or phencyclidine, is a dissociative anesthetic, which means that it causes a patient undergoing surgery to be oblivious of physical pain. Because of problems with severe behavioral reactions to PCP, it was restricted to veterinary use. But it is easily manufactured in illegal laboratories, which is the main source of street supplies.

PCP is included in the section on hallucinogens because its effects include distortions in perception and judgment, but it differs from the other hallucinogens in some respects. Laboratory animals demonstrate that PCP is highly reinforcing and therefore highly addictive. PCP causes a psychotic state that can persist for prolonged periods of time and is indistinguishable clinically from schizophrenia. It also causes agitation and aggressive behavior, sometimes to an extreme degree. PCP is known on the street as "angel dust" and is sometimes sold to unsuspecting users as THC (the active ingredient in marijuana) or is laced into poor-quality marijuana to increase its street value.

Addiction to PCP resembles crack addiction. Addicts use it in runs that may last for days, and then they crash. The drug causes profound stimulation of the brain and can cause nystagmus (rhythmic jerking movements of the eye), muscular rigidity, and seizures, as well as high fevers, sharp increases in blood pressure, and destruction of muscle tissue.

There are a number of other hallucinogens with differing properties and durations of action. The indole-type hallucinogens have chemical structures resembling the neurotransmitter serotonin, and are so named because they contain a chemical component known as an indole ring. They include the ergot alkaloids. LSD, DMT, and psilocybin (found in some mushrooms) are indole-type hallucinogens. The phenylethyamines resemble the neurotransmitter norepinephrine and have stimulant qualities. Mescaline, DOM, MDA, and MDMA are phenylethylamine-type hallucinogens. MDA and MDMA belong to the class called "designer drugs," since they were specifically designed by chemists to have hallucinogenic properties. Illicit labs have produced many chemical variations of MDA and MDMA, which are untested and unsafe but often sold on the street with the Ecstasy label.

Like LSD, MDMA was studied extensively for possible uses in the field of psychiatry. The discovery that both MDA and MDMA have toxic actions on brain cells has limited their potential for legitimate use. These drugs have been shown to kill brain cells that produce serotonin. The long-term effect on users is not yet known, but it's feared that abnormalities in the serotoninergic systems of the brain will emerge over time in former users of these drugs. Since serotonin is important in the processing and control of emotions, these effects could be profound.

Hallucinogens cause changes in perception and cognition, with effects differing slightly among the different ones. The stimulant hallucinogens have additional effects similar to those of amphetamines. The addictiveness of the hallucinogens also varies. MDA and MDMA have been shown to cause laboratory animals to self-administer the drug, but pure LSD does not possess this quality. This indicates that MDA and MDMA interact in a reinforcing fashion in the pleasure center of the brain, as do drugs like amphetamines, cocaine, alcohol, and opiates.

The addictive use of hallucinogens alone is occasionally seen, but it occurs most commonly in people with multiple drug dependencies, who will use anything available to alter mood. People recovering from the abuse of hallucinogens sometimes experience flashbacks, or sudden hallucinatory experiences that mimic the effect of the drug. The cause of flashbacks is unclear. They can occur months to years after the drug is out of the system but usually fade with time.

### Inhalants

The inhalants are a diverse group of substances that include volatile liquids and anesthetic gasses. Among them are gasoline and petroleum derivatives, toluene, acetone, methyl butyl ketone, nitrous oxide, ether, chloroform, trichloromethane, tricloroethane, and alcoholic solvents.

Inhalants are readily available commercially, and are found in many industrial settings. Spray paint, correction fluid, airplane glue, and waterproofing sprays are some of the more common compounds that can be found in any discount store. Nitrous oxide is used as a refrigerant and as a propellant for whipping cream in the food service industry. It is also used in dental offices, where it is known as "laughing gas," and is commonly used for surgical anesthesia.

Inhalants cause an immediate high which lasts for a brief period of time and is often followed by a headache or nausea. The effect is similar to intoxication with alcohol, progressing from initial excitation and disinhibition to stupor and drowsiness after repeated inhalations.

Because they are cheap and easily obtained, inhalants are often abused by children and young teenagers. Inhalant abuse is also seen in rural and poverty-stricken areas. Native American and Hispanic youth are at particular risk. The abuse of nitrous oxide and volatile nitrates such as butyl and amyl nitrate are seen in more affluent adult populations.

The main problem with inhalants is toxicity. Short-term toxic effects include asphyxiation during inhalation and sudden cardiac arrhythmia. High doses of some inhalants can cause confusion, delirium, or pulmonary edema.

Long-term toxic effects include inflammation of the brain and degeneration of nerves both within the brain and in the sensory and motor nerves of the body. Damage to the kidney, liver, and lungs can occur. Degeneration of muscle tissue may take place, as well as damage to the part of the brain that controls balance and coordination. Loss of intellectual functioning (dementia) may also result from the use of some substances.

Inhalant abusers seen in treatment settings often manifest severe problems with judgment and personality. Abuse of and dependence on multiple substances, including alcohol, marijuana, and cocaine, is also frequently seen. Since the pattern of abusing inhalants often begins at a young age, these people are frequently profoundly deficient in social skills. Addicts who begin in childhood miss out on the performance of many important developmental tasks.

# 5. The Course of Addictive Disease

Most people who start drinking or using drugs do not intend to become alcoholics or drug addicts. How does it happen?

At least half of all the people who develop addiction carry genes that make them more vulnerable to the condition. But it's not simply genetics. A combination of factors must come together in order for addiction to occur.

First, the substance has to be available, and you have to have some willingness to try it. If your family drinks or does drugs, then you are more likely to see this as normal behavior, as something adults do. Most of the patients I've treated in hospital settings for addiction started out with beer or marijuana on the weekends with friends. Drug prevention campaigns in the schools aim at nipping this kind of behavior in the bud, which is a good idea but hard to accomplish given a social climate that encourages drinking and drug use.

The future addict finds that drinking or using drugs solves some psychological or emotional problems. For many, it eases the shyness and awkwardness of socializing. If you already have problems with depression or anxiety, you may find temporary relief with alcohol or marijuana. Or your journey might start with prescription medications for pain or anxiety. In any case, you learn that you can find relief from uncomfortable feelings when you're high.

Many addicts, especially women, have experienced psychological trauma and various types of abuse. Being intoxicated or high lends a feeling of well-being and provides an escape from the psychological effects of the trauma.

It's at this point that casual or recreational use slips into reliance on the drug for its emotional effects. You remember the pleasurable experience of being high and don't see that many negative consequences, so you try to repeat the experience. Obtaining the drug, using it, and recovering from its effects begins to become a priority. You have now drifted over into substance abuse.

At this stage, most people ignore the possibility that addiction could develop. This is the beginning of denial. You might tell yourself, "I can control it." Or you might latch on to some misinformation that allows you to minimize the risks: "Marijuana is only psychologically addicting" or "They are just trying to scare kids away from using drugs." You may have an inaccurate idea of what an alcoholic or an addict is, and decide that as long as you can keep a job, don't get violent, and don't crave the substance all the time, you are not really addicted.

### Denial

I never cease to be amazed at how certain some people are that they are not addicted to a substance. But I also understand that this is a typical and important symptom of addiction. It is what we call denial.

Denial is an unconscious defense mechanism. Defense mechanisms are an important part of the psyche; they operate to keep us on an even keel emotionally and to protect our self-esteem. We all use them. Two examples are repression, which allows us to exclude painful or conflicted memories from our consciousness, and sublimation, which allows us to act out unconscious fantasies in socially useful ways. And there are many more.

Denial is seen in a variety of circumstances but occurs in a specialized form in addiction. Basically, a person in denial continues to maintain that an obvious reality is not true. While addiction is developing, the user desperately wants to continue to manage moods with a substance. It's like getting caught between a rock and a hard place. On the one hand, you probably know a lot about the particular dangers of your drug of choice, be it alcohol, marijuana, cocaine, or something else. But on the other hand, you cannot envision living life without the option of changing your mood. You might fear that you could never again enjoy socializing or that you would become overwhelmed by depression or anxiety. You might bury such a fear so deeply that you don't even know it's there. But you have a persistent feeling of hopelessness about ever being able to stop using. One way to manage this inner conflict is to slowly but steadily distort your perception of reality so that you can convince yourself that it is okay to continue using. This is denial.

"I can quit any time I want to" is denial in a nutshell. "I can quit" is a denial of the reality of the addiction; "any time I want to" is a rationalization. It is an example of the dishonesty that creeps in as addiction develops. The truth of the matter is that you really don't want to *quit*. You are addicted. You may want to learn how to drink or use drugs and avoid the negative consequences, but you don't want to quit. The addiction is serving a lot of important psychological functions at this point and giving it up involves changing the way you live.

Denial can be subtle or extreme. The longer the addiction is present and the more severe the consequences, the stronger it gets. I interviewed a man at a treatment center who had had five DUI arrests, had lost his job and family, and had been ordered by the court to get treatment. Our conversation went something like this:

> *It says here in the chart that you have had over five DUI arrests. Is that correct?*
> Oh, yeah [laughing]. And they've picked me up for public drunk, too. Probably five or six times.
> *I see. Did you lose your job because of your drinking?*
> No. They let me go because I was late for work.

*But you were late because you were hung over?*
Yeah.
*Your wife left you last year. She has sole custody of the kids, right?*
Yeah. I can see them with the social worker. But I don't want to.
They don't care about me anyhow.
*She left because of your drinking?*
[Angry] No! That woman left me because she's a control freak,
and I'm not about ready to let any woman control me.
*So none of these things have to do with your drinking except the
DUIs and the public drunks?*
Nope. And just because you get a DUI doesn't mean you're
an alcoholic. Heck, anyone could get a DUI the way things are
today.
*You're not an alcoholic?*
No, ma'am.
*So what are you doing here in a treatment center?*
Look. I'm just here because my lawyer told me the judge would
go easy if I went to treatment. You know, I'll have to do jail time
for this last DUI.
*Yes, I know that. Do you think it might be wise to stop drinking?*
I can stop. I'm not an alcoholic.

Denial separates the awareness that a negative consequence
has occurred from the emotional impact it should have. In
order to accomplish this, you begin to place blame outside
yourself. It wasn't your drinking too much at the bar that
resulted in the DUI; it was the overzealous cops. It wasn't
your being hung over or undependable that made the boss
upset; the boss was being unreasonable and demanding.

Smoking is a good example. There has been a massive
publicity campaign in recent years to educate the public
about the dangers of smoking. But a smoker who is confronted with the health risks is likely to say, "Gotta die somehow. Might as well die happy." This really isn't slow suicide,
as some people believe. It is denial.

## Some Words for the Addict

You may have begun to use alcohol or drugs because of the temporary relief you got from emotional discomfort. But there comes a point when the drug takes over and through its effects on the brain becomes its own motivation for continuing use. At this point, addiction—with the associated changes in brain functioning—has occurred. There is no way to tell exactly when this happens, but once it does the addict has another dilemma. What used to be a handy tool now becomes a heavy burden. One cocaine addict put it this way: "I was spending a hundred dollars just to feel nervous for fifteen minutes. But I couldn't stop." The drug wasn't doing what it was supposed to do any more, but *not* using was no longer a choice. The inner drive to use has little to do with the reason you started.

What has happened is that your brain has learned that the drug produces pleasure. The pleasure center in the brain sends strong signals to other parts of the brain and motivates you to use again. Once this has occurred, your choices about drug use become more and more irrational. This powerful effect reinforces the denial mechanism. The personality starts to change as your basic goal in life becomes supporting and continuing the addiction.

You become more and more self-centered. As your main interest in life becomes supporting the addiction, other activities become less important. You might skip social events if they don't provide an opportunity to drink or get high. You begin to choose friends based on whether or not they drink or use drugs. If you're hung over on a Monday morning, you might call in sick to work.

Typically you will not see the ways in which your drinking or drug use interferes with relationships. When arguments occur about your behavior, you defensively blame the other person instead of looking at yourself. When you're intoxicated, you are more likely to act on feelings of resentment, which leads to fights. The emotional needs of the people around you become less important, and you may find yourself resenting your spouse or children because they seem demanding. Having given the addiction the highest priority, you have no problem with diverting funds to support it, regardless of other necessities. This leads to more fights and more resentment.

Some people are able to maintain a modicum of functioning while continuing their addiction. You might control your behavior just enough so that you can avoid some consequences. For example, you might be able to keep your job and avoid legal difficulties. But it is likely that your relationships are suffering and that you are not realizing your potential for achievement. You are also risking the physical complications of your addiction, such as cirrhosis with alcohol or lung damage with marijuana.

While all this is going on, the spiritual life is suffering as well. A person's relationship with God goes on the back burner along with all other relationships. Religious teachings and moral imperatives become relative rather than absolute. This allows the addict to continue without experiencing guilt. Many people develop resentments toward God. This might be because of something terrible that happened or it might be the consequence of a consistent turning away from God. In any case, by the time the addiction is full blown you are spiritually bankrupt.

A moral deterioration also occurs while the addiction is progressing. This can be striking in the case of strongly addictive drugs like crack cocaine. People find themselves selling cherished personal belongings, going through savings accounts, stealing from family members, shoplifting, trading sex for drugs, or becoming entrenched in a criminal underground.

You become caught in a cycle of denial, rationalization, and justification. You might have a bit of insight; in quiet moments, you might suspect that the addiction is not worth the price. But when the motivation to use again kicks in, this voice is stilled. Everyone else becomes the enemy—the angry spouse or parent, the "narcs," the straight-laced church people, the unreasonable boss. The addiction has created an illusory world in which it is the number-one priority. The reason you started using has disappeared, and the temporary relief the substance gave you has long since diminished.

You are stuck with whatever the original problem was—shyness, anxiety, depression, abuse—and now you have more problems piling up as your world collides with reality. Relationships break down, jobs are lost, financial problems build, and you may have trouble with the law as well as physical problems caused by the addictive substance.

A housewife who started drinking at night to get to sleep finds that she cannot sleep at all, despite drinking continuously all evening. A trucker who began using amphetamines to stay awake during long hauls finds that he can't keep his weight up, that he is paranoid and restless, and that his skin is breaking out in sores. A college student who started using marijuana to relax at parties finds that he can't get through the day without smoking, that he is coughing all the time, and that he is failing in school.

During the time that this downward spiral is occurring, you are probably making some attempts to control it. You might adopt various rules—no hard liquor, only beer. No drinking before five p.m. on workdays. Drinking only on the weekends. No more crack, only marijuana. No more than fifty dollars per week on drugs.

You might even stop drinking or using for prolonged periods of time. But because you haven't addressed the other issues, this attempt will eventually fail. You are attacking the symptom—the use of the substance—without looking at the cause, which is the addictive disease itself with all its different aspects.

A "dry drunk" is an alcoholic who has stopped drinking because of the negative consequences but has never looked at the damage that has occurred to relationships, personality, and morals. If you're in this situation, you are probably miserable. Addiction professionals call this "white knuckling," because it's as though you're holding on so hard to keep yourself from using that your knuckles get white. And eventually you get tired. It's at this point that addicts often switch their drug of choice, from alcohol to marijuana or benzodiazepines, from opiates to alcohol, from cocaine to crystal meth, and so on.

If you manage to stay dry and not relapse or switch substances, you still suffer from the distortions in thinking and the damage to relationships that developed as the addiction progressed. You probably continue to place blame elsewhere for your shortcomings and to be self-centered and insensitive to the needs of others. Your self-esteem and sense of realistic effectiveness have been damaged by the addiction. As one recovering alcoholic put it, "I'm not going to be a dry drunk, because I can be just as unhappy drinking."

Where is this spiral leading? Remember the lab rats who are given a choice between food pellets and cocaine. They will press the lever for the cocaine, despite their need for food, until they collapse and die. Even self-preservation takes a backseat to the addiction. "I knew that I was either going to stay messed up, get locked up, or get covered up," said one woman at a treatment center. That is the truth about addiction. You might be able to continue to control environment and consequences for a while, but eventually your quality of life suffers, and the outcome may even be death.

In some ways people with more destructive addictions are fortunate, because consequences are severe and obvious and the dreadful possibilities are laid out before them over and over again. People who experience less dramatic consequences might continue using or drinking all their lives without ever facing the need to recover. But their relationships wither and their spiritual life fades away.

The choice is this: recovery or death. Addictive disease is

a fatal illness, with no cure. There is a chance for a reprieve. Addiction can be brought into remission, and the addict can begin repairing the damage and rebuilding his or her life. But addiction is the only fatal illness I know of that contains an element of will. The addict is the one who chooses the outcome. Addicts in recovery choose their outcome every day, and so do active addicts. With every day that goes by, you have the choice: addiction or recovery.

Recovering addicts describe this as an elevator going down. The bottom floor is death. You can get off the elevator at any floor you choose, or you can ride it all the way down. It's your decision, and yours alone.

### Some Words for the Family Member

We will now take a look at what happens to those who care about the person developing an addiction. (In the next chapter we will examine more closely the effects of addiction on the family.)

The refrain of a country song goes like this: "Whiskey, if you were a woman . . ." The singer laments the fact that she has to compete with whiskey for her husband's affections. If you are in a relationship with someone who is addicted, you are in a love triangle. We have just seen that, as the addiction progresses, the addict's priorities change so that the addiction is at the center of the person's life. When this happens, the addict is no longer able to provide affection and support, at least not in a consistent fashion. So you, as the loved one, are left to fend for yourself, more or less, in getting your emotional needs met.

If you grew up in a family where one or both of your parents was addicted, or if there is a lot of addiction in your extended family, you might not notice that this is a problem. You would have come of age in a situation where it was "normal" to expect that others' emotional needs were not recognized, and a relationship with someone who is addicted is familiar to you, even if it is stressful.

But at the same time that the addict is becoming more focused on the addiction, and less on you and your needs, he or she is also becoming more dependent on your support. This is where a great deal of complex emotional game playing comes in.

Addicts are often fun-loving, friendly, warm, and engaging people when they are not drinking or using drugs. If you fell in love with someone who was addicted, or who has since developed an addiction, don't kick yourself too hard. You didn't cause it, and the addict certainly didn't expect it to happen. But you should understand that as long as the addiction is active and the addict is not in recovery, you are dealing with a different person, one whose primary motivation in life is the maintenance of the addiction, not of the relationship.

Even though the addict's number-one priority is the addiction, the relationship with you will also become important, but not in a healthy way. Your interest in and love for the addict becomes an important tool. You are available to provide emotional and financial support, excuses, even bail money. Because your emotional needs are not being met, you may come to believe that giving in to the addict's needs and demands is a reasonable substitute, while you continue to hold out hope that things will change.

You may learn to give in order to get. In fact, this may be a primary way of getting your emotional needs met if you grew up in an addicted family. When you see a person with a problem of some type and believe that you can be of some use, you are ready and willing to "help." This meets your need for attention and emotional attachment in a superficial way, but it is a second-rate substitute. This is the coping strategy that we call codependency.

As the addiction progresses, your giving will increase, and so will the addict's demands and dysfunctional behavior. While this is happening, you are likely to become angry.

You will get frustrated because things are not changing. The person is not responding to your demand that something be done about the addiction, and you are getting tired of endless disappointments and broken promises.

You may become depressed. In an atmosphere of continuous emotional deprivation, you may begin to believe that you are not worthy of love and attention. You feel unable to change your situation, and you may begin to feel hopeless about things ever being different.

If the addict is emotionally or physically abusive, you may also begin to have a sense of guilt and shame as a result of the abuse. If your self-esteem was already shaky before you entered the relationship, as is often the case with those who grew up in an addicted family, it now begins to take a free fall. But the more your self-esteem falls, the more likely you are to become further engaged in the game playing that allows the addiction to continue.

The insecurity and unpredictability of living with an addict leads to an emphasis on control. As the addiction gets more out of hand, you become more focused on maintaining control. Initially, this centers around the addict's behavior. If you could just control the supply of alcohol or the amount of spending money or could keep tabs at all times on the addict's whereabouts, then maybe things would change for the better. But after a while a new dynamic appears in the relationship. You are criticized for being controlling, for not trusting, and for damaging the relationship. Your self-esteem falls further, and the addict has another excuse to use.

Of course, what is really controlling the whole relationship is the addiction itself. But this is difficult to see because of the subtle way in which the situation develops.

Since it is impossible to control the addict or the addiction, you might attempt to gain a sense of control in other settings and with other relationships, perhaps becoming overly intrusive regarding family members or coworkers. Any kind of ambiguity provokes anxiety, so you cannot relax until you have things under control. This often leads to conflict, and, since controlling people and situations is generally impossible, you become exhausted and overwhelmed from the effort. You may feel like the mythical character in Hades whose task is to roll a boulder up a hill; every time he nears the top the boulder rolls back down.

Because of the conflict and the negative consequences resulting from the addiction, relationships often break up. You may finally become so unhappy that you leave, or the relationship may become abusive and you have to get away to be safe. If this is the case, it is important to remember that the effects of the addiction on your self-esteem, your coping strategies, and your way of relating to people will come with you. You will need to focus on your own recovery even if you leave the relationship.

Either way—whether you stay or leave—you will benefit from treatment and counseling for the effects the addiction has had on you. You will need to learn how to identify feelings accurately, how to get rid of the anger, how to assert yourself so as to get your emotional needs met, how to trust again, and how to release your urge to control the world around you.

Family members of addicts often develop their own problems with addiction. Eating disorders, such as compulsive overeating, are common in family members of addicts. It is also easy for family members to begin using drugs or alcohol to cope with the pain of dealing with an addict and to become addicted themselves. This is especially true if there is a family history of addiction and therefore a genetic susceptibility.

### Recovery or Death?

There may be no cure for addiction, but there are ways of bringing it into remission. Let's look at how people approach major changes, such as those involved in recovery. Prochaska and DeClemente studied this process in detail, and found that people who are making significant changes in lifestyle go through the following stages: precontemplation, contemplation, action, and maintenance or relapse.

When you are in the precontemplation phase, you are basically enjoying the addiction and do not consider that it might be necessary to change. You are in full denial and able to successfully fend off any anxiety about the addiction. As negative consequences increase, you may begin to wonder if you might be better off quitting. But you are able to mobilize various strategies, such as blaming, projection, rationalization, and justification, to continue to feel comfortable about your addiction. If someone challenges you about your drinking or drug use, you have a ready reply. In fact, if certain people, such as your spouse or parents, approach you on the subject, you become more determined to persist.

When you enter the contemplation stage, you are beginning to wonder if you need to make some changes. You may not completely accept that the alcohol or drug use has to stop entirely, but you are beginning to recognize that some of your problems might be a result of the addiction. You may sense a loss of control over the use of the substance, and you may realize that it is no longer providing you with relief from uncomfortable feelings.

At this point, the types of interactions that you have with your family or with treatment professionals can either move you along towards taking some action or push you back into the precontemplation stage. It's as if you are on a seesaw, with part of you wanting to continue the addiction and part of you wanting to stop. If someone else sits on one side of the seesaw—for example, by criticizing you aggressively for the addiction—you may become anxious and then angry, and go on drinking or using for a while before you again feel comfortable enough to consider changing.

(Family members should understand the importance of

this stage. They can facilitate and support the addict getting treatment and entering recovery, but if they remain locked in a battle for control they will be making it more difficult. In Al-Anon and other 12-step programs for family members, the principle of "loving detachment" is taught. Loved ones accept that they cannot control what the addict does about the addiction and become detached by giving up their wish for such control. They remain supportive of any attempts at recovery but do not bail the addict out of difficult situations.)

In the action phase, you make a decision to do something about the addiction. Now you need two things: a belief that it is possible to recover and a way to get started.

It's useful at this point to go to a 12-step meeting. You can find an Alcoholics Anonymous meeting or a Narcotics Anonymous meeting by looking in the phone book. Alcoholics Anonymous is usually listed on the first page. Many cities have branch offices of the National Council on Alcoholism and Drug Dependence where you can also find lists of local meetings. The local mental health center usually has such information, and meetings are often listed in the local paper.

You don't have to make a decision about recovery in order to go to a meeting. According to the preamble that is recited at the beginning of most AA meetings, "The only requirement for membership is a desire to stop drinking." All you need is the desire. You don't have to talk, and you probably shouldn't at first, except to introduce yourself. It's important to listen to others who are further along in recovery. If you want to talk one-on-one with someone who is recovering, just ask; most members are more than willing. Talking with people who have been where you are now and are living happy and productive lives in recovery helps you believe that it is possible for you.

You may need treatment in an alcohol and drug facility. Private and public facilities are usually listed in the yellow pages of the phone book. Many government-funded programs are available for those who do not have the money for a private facility. You can often find out about these by calling your local mental health center.

Treatment centers serve several important functions. They can help you get through a period of medical detoxification and address any crises that have arisen because of the consequences of your addiction. But, as we've learned, stopping the use of the alcohol or drugs is only a minor part of recovery. Treatment centers can assist you in developing the coping skills and self-awareness that you need to stay in recovery for the long term, after you leave the facility. Most treatment centers make use of the principles of 12-step recovery and encourage your participation in AA or similar groups after discharge. Treatment centers also work with family members to help them learn about what is involved in recovery and deal with the broader effects of the addiction.

At the next stage in the process of change is a fork in the road. You will either maintain the changes you have made and continue to grow, or you will relapse and return to the addiction.

Maintenance involves a process of continuing growth and self-awareness. As your life gets back on track, you may discover that there are issues that need to be addressed. Remember that many people begin drinking or using drugs in order to avoid painful feelings. You may have had a troubled childhood or you may suffer from anxiety or depression. These problems have to be faced in an ongoing fashion. The trick here is keeping your eye on the ball. Addiction is never cured, but it can go into remission. To maintain remission, you have to take care of yourself and continue doing those things that have kept you sober so far.

Relapse is a continuous risk. Many people relapse during the first two years or so of sobriety, but a surprisingly large number also relapse after five, ten, or twenty years. One type of relapse involves the development of another addiction, or cross-addiction (see chapter 3). People who have overcome an addiction to cocaine, for example, may get in trouble with alcohol later on. Behavioral addictions, such as gambling, overeating, or compulsive sexual behavior, sometimes crop up as well. If you go back and trace the course of early recovery for those people, you often find that the emotional, psychological, and spiritual aspects of the addiction were not completely addressed. They have been "white knuckling" and continue to have problems coping with painful emotions.

Does everyone who is addicted eventually get into recovery? Sadly, no. Outcome measures—surveys that track the success of people in recovery—tell us that 5 to 60 percent stay sober over the long term. These studies use somewhat different criteria and have different durations, but we do know that some behaviors will improve a person's chances of staying sober: consistent attendance at 12-step and aftercare meetings, willingness to reenter treatment if relapse occurs, and active involvement by the family in a recovery program and aftercare.

It's important to remember that there is an element of will involved in the disease of addiction. If you are willing, if you remain open to suggestions, and if you try to be thoroughly honest with yourself, you can make it.

# 6. Addiction and the Family

"Addiction is a family disease." This observation is commonly made in addiction treatment circles, but what does it mean? Exactly how does addiction affect the family?

The statement does not mean that families are responsible for the addiction; the addict makes his or her own choices. However, as the addiction progresses, a number of dysfunctional patterns typically occur in the addict's family. These patterns may lead to self-defeating behaviors and interactions that can interfere with recovery, despite the family's best intentions. And as long as the addict suffers, the entire family suffers. This is why addiction professionals consider treatment of the family to be an integral part of the treatment of addiction.

The effects of addiction on the family are widespread. About one out of three people in the United States has a relative with a substance abuse problem. For one out of four, it is a close relative (mother, father, sibling, or child). When we look at the families of alcoholics and addicts, we see a marked increase in divorce, domestic violence, child abuse, depression, anxiety, and general medical problems. Spouses of addicts tend to be more depressed than their peers and to have more medical complaints. Children raised in families with addicts exhibit a range of problems: poor conduct and academic achievement, delinquency, low self-esteem and depression. Adults who grew up in such families suffer from depression and social anxiety and have difficulty in relationships. This can be the case even if the addicted family member belonged to a previous generation.

We know that if the addict and the family get into recovery, many of the effects on the family begin to diminish within a couple of years. But it is often the family itself that unwittingly interferes with the process of recovery. Active participation in the companion 12-step programs such as Al-Anon and Narc-Anon, family therapy, or individual counseling help to move the entire family along the path of recovery and to eliminate some of the unseen resistance.

### The Healthy Family

To understand the addict's family, let's first look at families in general and how they function. In its most basic form, a family is a task-oriented group, with the primary purpose being the promotion of the health and welfare of its members. Although families may be made up of any combination of members in relationship to one another, let's look at a family that consists of two parents and several children living in the same house; the father is the primary wage earner, and the mother has primary responsibility for the day-to-day care of the children.

Roles in this family are clearly defined and mutually agreed upon. They are age-appropriate, with clear patterns of communication and clear boundaries. The parents have a healthy, mature relationship, and their emotional needs are met by each other or by other adults. They are therefore able to tune into and respond to the emotional needs of the children without having to take into account their own needs. The children's role is to get educated and grow up. They do not have to be concerned about their parents' well-being; it is a one-way relationship. There is a healthy intergenerational boundary.

By the same token, parents and children alike in this family allow each other to express themselves, to work out their own problems, and to have privacy. There are healthy interpersonal boundaries. Family members are free to experience and express the entire range of emotions that define their experiences in life, good or bad. They are free to pursue goals and interests outside the family, to be creative, and to give of themselves to others in the community.

There are three things to notice about this family: (1) it has a distinct task—raising the kids—that everyone agrees upon, (2) it has a well-defined and healthy structure that is geared toward completing the task, and (3) it has efficient ways of dealing with feelings and identifying and communicating physical and emotional needs. Because those elements are in place in the family, its members experience the home as a relaxing and renewing place to be, and they are therefore able to go out into the world as creative and productive beings. Furthermore, when crises such as illness, death, or financial setbacks come up, the mechanisms are in place to deal with these additional pressures without straining the family to the breaking point.

Another phenomenon that we see in all types of families, as well as in many biological and sociological systems, is that of homeostasis, which means "staying the same." Biological systems tend to stay the same, because homeostatic mechanisms keep them that way. For example, our body temperature generally stays about the same. If we become too hot, we sweat and cool off. If we become too cold, we shiver and warm up. On a psychological and emotional level the same principle applies. We tend to resist change. Sometimes choices that may at first seem self-defeating can be understood if we realize that the person making them was just trying to keep things on an even keel, consciously or unconsciously. Families also will resist change and will adapt in a variety of ways to any stresses that threaten to change the status quo. Sometimes these ways are helpful, but sometimes they are not.

While the family is trying to cope with the addiction, a lot of the changes that are made serve to keep the situation as stable as possible. In a family with someone who is recovering, there will also be a general resistance to change for the same reason. Anything that is different—whether it's positive or negative—will be hard to incorporate into the family system if for no other reason than that it rocks the boat, which is uncomfortable.

## The Addicted Family

Let's contrast the family described above with one that is dealing with addiction. This family is also task oriented, but the primary task is different—it is no longer the promotion of the emotional growth and well-being of its members but has become one of dealing with the addiction and coping with the consequences of the addict's behavior.

To this end, a number of mechanisms develop. While the addict is trying to manipulate the family so that he or she can continue to use alcohol or drugs, the family is trying to manipulate the addict into stopping. The addiction has taken center stage, but the other tasks, such as raising children, making a living, and meeting physical and emotional needs, are still important and must be tended to somehow. The family develops a variety of ways of completing necessary tasks while being taxed by the addiction. But because addiction stresses the family's emotional resources, members often compromise by putting aside what appear to be less important needs in order to meet more pressing ones. These compromises lead to what addiction professionals call dysfunctional patterns of interaction.

The term "dysfunctional," though, should be be seen in the proper perspective. The ways in which various families cope with addiction are so similar that one wonders whether this is a "normal" way for a group or a family to adapt to the presence of an addiction. The dysfunctional nature of the patterns and coping skills tends to become more apparent when individuals raised in addicted families attempt to function in other settings, such as at school, on the job, or in relationships outside the immediate family. It is in those situations that the impairment in emotional and interpersonal functioning becomes most apparent.

The specific manifestations of the dysfunction in the addicted family depend on the circumstances even if the overall patterns are similar. Those circumstances might include the position of the addict in the family (spouse, parent, child), whether or not there is abusive behavior, how vital the addict's role is in the overall functioning of the family, and outside resources the family can use in adapting to the addiction. In some families the dysfunction is subtle and in others it is quite blatant.

Nonetheless, there are some characteristics that are common to most addicted families. These include denial of the addiction and an emphasis on the appearance of normality to outsiders; a tendency to assign and displace blame; an unspoken ban on the expression of strong negative emotions, especially anger; conflict about how to deal with the addict's behavior, which may split the family into factions; problems with boundaries in relationships and between generations; difficulties with trust and intimacy; and the adoption of characteristic roles that reflect the pathological demands imposed by the addiction.

### Denial of the Situation

The addict's behavior is often embarrassing and leads to embarrassing consequences, such as encounters with the law, lost jobs, or social ostracism. As we have seen, the addict develops a system of denial that allows for a disconnection between the memory of a negative consequence and the associated emotion. The family does much the same thing. For all the turmoil caused by the family's frantic attempts to control the addiction, members also try their best to maintain appearances, to put their best foot forward. In the face of the addict's deteriorating behavior, families will go to great lengths to minimize and justify the situation and to present a positive image to the outside world. This is a family with a secret, and with a secret comes deception.

Facing the truth about the addiction is often just too painful. That would be the healthiest course of action in the long run, but it is not the one that many families take at first. What develops instead is an unspoken agreement that the truth about the addiction will not be discussed or revealed to outsiders. In some families this deception becomes so pervasive that family members themselves are unable to perceive that the addiction exists, and they proceed with life as though it is not present at all.

But one of the consequences of building a system of denial is that the family has to deal with the frequent crises that accompany addiction while ignoring a large chunk of reality—that of the addiction itself. If the alcoholic father loses his job, the family does not permit itself to recognize that it was because of the addiction to alcohol. It has to be someone else's fault. Enormous effort is sometimes expended on the wrong problem, while the family system continues to move toward disaster. It's not unlike what happened when the captain of the *Titanic* chose to ignore the icebergs.

### Blaming

Blaming is a symptom of the problem. Identifying the addiction as the cause of a particular difficulty means admitting that the addiction is present. But doing that risks revealing the secret that there is serious trouble in the family. So family members find others to blame when things go wrong. Parents blame the school system when their addicted teenager flunks out of school. The alcoholic blames the nagging spouse when a relapse occurs. One person in the divorce blames the other when the real reason that the marriage failed was addiction.

Parents send their addicted young adult child to psychiatrist after psychiatrist in an effort to cure the "chemical imbalance" that they believe has caused the addiction.

### The "Don't Talk" Rule

Blaming is also a symptom of the ban that is placed on strong negative emotions. Addiction professionals refer to this as the "don't talk/don't feel" rule; it is another way in which the family adapts in an attempt to prevent the addiction from rocking the boat.

The "don't talk/don't feel" rule restricts what topics can be talked about and what emotions can be expressed. Eventually it restricts what emotions can be felt. It is not okay to openly discuss the father's escalating alcohol problem or the sister's drug problem. It is no longer permissible to be angry if something upsetting happens or sad if something bad happens or joyful if something great happens. All emotions are passed through a filter: if what you are feeling is consistent with the basic assumptions under which the family is operating, it is acceptable. Otherwise, you did not feel it.

The feeling and expression of anger are particularly distorted. In this type of family, it is not uncommon for hostile or angry behavior to be used mainly as a tool for manipulation rather than as the genuine expression of a feeling that could lead to a productive change in direction. Anger is also seen as dangerous because verbal or physical violence often occurs in addicted families. These families learn to walk on eggshells around the abusive person (who is often the addict, but not always). Family members may also be emotionally traumatized to the extent that even appropriate expressions of anger or conflict trigger anxiety and fear of upheaval or retaliation. Guilt-ridden addicts may wish to avoid any expression of conflict when they are not using the addictive substance. If a relapse occurs, a belief may develop in the family that stress or discord has triggered the addict's behavior. Therefore it is more important to keep the peace than to express one's true feelings.

Many different reasons and usually years of experience reinforce the "don't talk/don't feel" rule. But the problem with suppressing strong negative emotions is that all other emotions are also suppressed. It's like trying to avoid seeing the color red—the only way to do so is to close your eyes and see no colors at all. Members of addicted families have a great deal of difficulty correctly identifying feeling states, and especially identifying the many subtle nuances of different feelings. Feelings and emotions begin to fall into two basic categories—okay and upset. Anger is often mistaken for anxiety or stress. Depression and sadness are experienced as irritability. This is a serious problem in the long run for all members of the family.

Our feelings and emotions help us navigate through relationships and situations. Like the sonar system in a submarine, we send out emotional signals, and we receive feedback which tells us in what direction to proceed. If the sensitivity of the system is damaged because of a "don't talk/don't feel" rule, then it won't be long before some type of interpersonal catastrophe occurs—a relationship on the rocks, a personality conflict at work, or other problems of coping.

### Splits

As the addiction spirals out of control, the family attempts to regain equilibrium in any way possible. The addict is busy obtaining and using the addictive substance and recovering from the results. The family is busy with damage control and with trying to prevent the addict from continuing. As we have seen, loss of control over the use of the substance is part of the definition of addiction. So we can imagine that the family's efforts to control the addiction are likely to fail. Nonetheless, almost every family will try.

In the process of trying to control the addiction, two

schools of thought will emerge in most families. Some people react to the threat of the family disintegrating, align with the addict's denial system, and then excuse, cover up, or attempt to compensate for the addiction. Others feel that the solution for both the addict and the family as a whole is to expel the addict from the family, cut off all resources, and force the addict to sink or swim. Of course, neither approach is likely to be successful in the long run, but the argument itself dissipates a good bit of tension in the family. It is an indirect but acceptable way of expressing negative feelings about the addict and his or her behavior.

On both sides, the basic assumption is the same—that it is possible, somehow, to find a way to control the addiction and fix the problem. People who have grown up in addicted families often respond to tension and conflict in outside situations by attempting to control others, and they may feel inappropriately responsible for the behaviors of others. Life in an addicted family is often unpredictable and chaotic, and this further reinforces the need that family members have to control others.

### Boundaries

When family members learn to deny reality, deflect blame, suppress emotions, and attempt to control the behavior of others, their relationships are profoundly affected. Healthy relationships have boundaries—a sense of where one's self ends and the other's begins. We can see, then, how boundaries become problematic for the addicted family. Blaming, for example, involves a blurring of personal responsibility. The "don't talk/don't feel" rule is a boundary invasion. It is an external force that dictates your personal thoughts and feelings. What you feel and what you can say about it is no longer a private matter, but is subject to the control and censorship of others.

Boundaries also exist between generations. In the healthy

family, there is a boundary between the parents as a couple and the children as a group. The parents discuss and experience some things that they do not share with the children and vice versa. These boundaries are one-directional. Certain things may be deliberately withheld from the children in order to protect them from stress and allow them to focus on their own growth and development. For example, while it is appropriate for a child's emotional needs to be brought to and met by the parents, it is not appropriate for the mother or father to come to the child with emotional needs, because that would burden the child, increase the child's anxiety level, and interfere with the child's development.

In the addicted family, the stress level is often so high that the children pick up on the parents' emotional distress and begin to feel responsible for fixing the family. It is not uncommon for at least one child, often the oldest, to assume the role of junior parent in order to relieve some of the pressure.

The parent-child roles may also be reversed. Children are exquisitely sensitive to emotional upset in the parents, and often a child will assume the role of emotional, or sometimes physical, caretaker for the addict or for another overburdened family member such as the addict's spouse. In both situations, the child's development is hampered. The child is forced to deny age-appropriate needs in the interest of the family's functioning and survival.

### Trust and Intimacy

In this family where boundaries shift, roles are reversed, emotions are censored, and tension, chaos, and unpredictability are part of daily life, it is almost impossible for family members to develop a solid sense of trust. People often do not do what they say they will do. Situations change abruptly and without apparent reason. The emotional climate of the home is never predictable, and much depends upon whether or not the addict has used the addictive substance.

Since emotions are suppressed or denied, family members are unable to accurately tune into one another's needs. They cannot be trusted to respond consistently or in understanding and empathic ways. In short, relationships are experienced as basically treacherous and stressful. It is no wonder that a person from an addicted family has difficulty experiencing intimacy with others.

### Roles

The power of addiction as a molding force in a family is illustrated by the observation made by many addiction professionals that certain stereotypical roles appear in the addicted family. The reason is that these roles are necessary in order for the family to continue on an even keel in the face of the addiction and the multitude of ways in which it distorts the way the family functions.

The chief role that is seen in most addicted families, including addicted couples, is that of the enabler. The enabler, often the spouse, gradually takes over the responsibilities that the addict is failing to assume. At the same time, there is an escalating effort to try to control the addict's behavior and return to the way life used to be, or to the way the enabler thinks it should be. But the enabler unwittingly allows the addiction to continue by protecting the addict from negative consequences. This is an entirely unintended result. The enabler's behavior is motivated by love for the addict and for the family and by a wish to help and to compensate for the addict's mistakes. But as the addiction progresses, as it inevitably will, the enabler gets caught in many impossible binds.

For example, the addict may be spending most of the weekly paycheck at the bar on the way home from work on Friday night. If the bills aren't paid, the lights and water eventually get turned off, and the family is evicted from the home. These negative consequences might motivate an addict to seek treatment. But while the addict is experiencing these negative consequences, the whole family is suffering as well. The enabler makes a logical choice and gets a job so that the bills will be paid despite the addict's behavior. This not only shields the addict from negative consequences but also protects the family as a whole.

The enabler may begin to resent the addict's irresponsibility, but, when anger is expressed directly, the addict's response is often to blame the enabler. "If you would get off my back I wouldn't need to drink" is an example. The more the enabler attempts to control the addict's behavior, the worse it gets, or so it seems. The addiction is actually going to progress with or without the enabler's help. But the enabler feels overly responsible, trapped, and increasingly angry, without the ability to express or sometimes even acknowledge that anger.

Roles that are frequently found among the children in an addicted family include the family hero (or banner carrier), the scapegoat, the lost child, and the mascot. Each of the roles serves to deflect and manage the high level of stress, tension, and anger that lies under the surface in addicted families.

The family hero, or banner carrier, is frequently the oldest child, and is a driven high achiever. This child, who often assumes the role of junior parent or caretaker, reassures the family, through public success, that things are still okay. The scapegoat, usually the second child, provides a ready target for blaming. Just as the family hero can do no wrong, the scapegoat can do no right. The lost child escapes the tension in the family by withdrawing into fantasy and will sometimes assume a caretaker role in order to merit attention. The mascot responds to the tension in the family by becoming the court jester but sacrifices the opportunity to be taken seriously and to be understood, especially when painful events take place.

These roles are consistently found in addicted families to a surprising degree, even across cultural and lifestyle lines. It is important to note, however, that a role often has little to do with the natural proclivities of the child playing it. The child responds to the stresses and forces within the addicted family system, and this shapes both behavior and self-concept. These children never learn to accurately identify emotional needs or develop a secure sense of self, and, as adults, are often highly sensitive to the emotional climate in a particular situation, but at the same time are unable to accurately sense inner emotions and needs. The concept of loving others and being loved is often understood at the level of meeting dependency needs rather than at the level of a true interest in the well-being of the other.

In other words, someone from this type of family will feel most secure in a relationship in which the other person has some kind of dependency need that allows for a sense of connectedness. When that dependency decreases, the relationship feels less secure, and anxiety levels go up. In a healthy relationship, on the other hand, increasing maturity and independence lead to a deepening of intimacy. From an emotional standpoint, people from addicted families are really marching to a different drummer. It's therefore not surprising that such people often end up marrying an addict or someone from an addicted family or a person with some type of emotional dependency.

In the mid-to-late 1980s, codependency was a popular topic in mental health circles. The concept of codependency arose from the study of the dynamics of the families of alcoholics and addicts, and contains the elements that we have discussed. Codependency is not a diagnosis in and of itself, but it is often found in the relational style of people who develop problems with depression and anxiety. It reflects a tendency to become emotionally invested in relationships with people who are not functioning independently, such as addicts. Although we generally think of the enabler as the one who is codependent, this style of relating is shared by all members of the addicted family, including the addict. In fact, it is not uncommon to see a reversal of roles once the addict enters recovery, with the addict now invested in the emotional dependency of the enabler.

With therapy, counseling, and time, family members can learn to become more sensitive to their own feelings and emotional needs. Once this occurs, it is possible for them to learn to tolerate more distance and emotional independence without undue anxiety and without needing to invade boundaries and attempt to exert control.

### Recovery

I decided to talk about recovery for families in this chapter, before the one on recovery for the addict, because the addict's family can provide one of the most critical support systems in the struggle for sobriety or one of the biggest obstacles.

While addiction is progressing in a family, an enormous amount of change is taking place, as we've seen. The family is struggling to stay together and keep on an even keel, while at the same time trying to "fix" the problems caused by the addicted member. The entanglements and manipulations that occur along the way are deeply entrenched.

Family members are often so exhausted and enraged by the time the addict enters treatment that no one in the family is willing to expend any further effort. They feel that it's time for the addict to shape up and take responsibility and for the treatment center to relieve them of some of the burden for a while. Blame gets shifted to the addict alone, and it's often hard for family members to become engaged in a therapy program just for themselves.

If you're at that point, or close to it, I'd like you to consider two things. Despite the frustration and anger, you're going to be much better off in the long run if you undertake your own recovery. Your active participation is helpful in many ways to the addict who is trying to recover, so you are promoting your desire to see the family's problems get "fixed." But, perhaps more important, you will probably find that there have been a number of ways in which the addiction has damaged your self-esteem, your sense of effectiveness as a person, your ability to trust, and your faith. *You* need some care. You have been taking care of everyone and everything else for a long time, and it's time for you to devote some effort to getting your own emotional needs met. Recovery will help with that.

I put this chapter before the next one for another reason as well. The addicted person doesn't always get better. In fact, there may be more losers than winners in this game. Addiction is a relapsing disorder, which means that some periods of abstinence may be followed by a return of the active addiction. It is difficult for people to get into a good program of sustained abstinence and long-term sobriety. You cannot bank on the addict getting better so that you can get better. The odds are it's not going to happen.

But you can recover from the damage and distortions that the addiction has caused in your life and in your family even if the addict is unable to achieve long-term sobriety.

### Facing the Problem

As we've seen, just as the addict develops denial while the addiction is progressing, families practice their own kind of denial, typically wishing to preserve a sense of normalcy and suppressing unpleasant feelings and realities. Although you can probably easily identify the addictive behavior as a problem—the addict's irresponsibility, dishonesty, unpredictability—you may have difficulty recognizing problems of your own that might be related to the addiction.

For example, you might be consistently engaging in rescuing behavior, not only of the addict when some crisis occurs but of everyone you care about, even in minor matters.

You may see this as being a caring and selfless person, and certainly you wouldn't be motivated to help if you weren't such a person to begin with. But what you're not seeing is that you are staving off anxiety and depression by becoming overinvolved in other people's problems; this is part of your denial.

You might simply be minimizing what's going on because it would be too painful to admit the full truth to yourself. Although you might be able to acknowledge that your loved one has had some "problems" with addiction, you don't see the necessity of doing everything that the drug counselor is suggesting. After all, the person isn't as bad off as some others you know of who are addicts.

This is a form of denial that is common to family members and addicts alike. Wise "old-timers" in AA and other 12-step programs address this line of thinking with one word—*yet*.

> Wife of an alcoholic at an open AA meeting: "My husband's drinking is not that bad. At least he hasn't had a DUI."
> Old-timer: "*Yet*."

The severity of the problem is not measured by the type of consequences. If it's addiction, it's severe. People who have been around addiction and recovery for a long time know that anything (bad) is possible if it has to do with the addiction and with the future.

Family members sometimes avoid recovery and minimize the addict's problems for another simple, but often overlooked, reason. They themselves may have a problem with addiction. This is not an uncommon situation. People who have grown up in families with addiction often unconsciously seek out a partner who has the same kind of problem. Addiction, as we've seen, has a strong genetic basis. So the spouse of an alcoholic, for example, may have a genetic vulnerability to alcoholism. We've noted that a permissive environment and psychological pain are both conducive to the development of addiction. It would be hard to find a better environment for the promotion of addiction than that of an addicted family.

Often the addictive behavior in the family member is disguised. The addiction might be to mood-altering prescription medication. Someone might have an eating disorder (very common in the families of addicts), be a compulsive gambler, or have a sexual addiction. These problems may be hidden under even more denial, and for a good reason. It's one thing to openly recognize that the addict, who is often getting center stage, has a problem. It's quite another to admit that the fallback person—the enabler on whom the family is depending—has one also. This person has the addiction in addition to being under enormous pressure to be fully functional, even overly functional at times. There's no *time* to deal with any more problems, or so it may seem. Unfortunately, things probably will not go well if the family is unable or unwilling to take the steps to face and then to work on these additional issues.

### Getting Better

Recovery for family members begins in much the same way that it begins for the addict. First, there must be an admission that there is a problem and a willingness to accept help. Next comes the discovery of just what the problem really is, followed by a gradual, lifelong learning process that leads to more effective coping and to emotional growth.

There are four principal avenues of treatment: education about addiction and recovery, group support, individual support, and psychiatric help.

#### EDUCATION

Educational materials not only provide you with information about what you are going through but help to normalize your experience and show you that you are not alone. Millions of people have been where you are right now, and there are probably hundreds in your area, or nearby, who are going through it at the present time. Feelings of guilt and shame usually run rampant in a dysfunctional family, and the simple knowledge that you are not bad, peculiar, or crazy can be very helpful.

Most alcohol and drug treatment centers provide an on-site educational program for family members. This usually includes videotapes and lectures given by a licensed addiction counselor who can answer questions and provide support. If you are not presently in contact with a treatment center, as is often the case, you can inquire at local centers to see if they provide a family program for people in the community who are living with an addict not currently in treatment. Some nationally based facilities that provide services for families can be found in appendix B of this book. Some useful books are listed there as well, along with Web sites of interest. Be a little leery of the Web sites if you are "surfing"; some are excellent, some are very informal, and some are misleading.

GROUP SUPPORT

Meeting regularly with a group of people who are in similar situations and developing long-term, supportive relationships is a *must* for family members. This usually entails devoting some evenings to 12-step meetings. You will have to find someone to watch the kids, get yourself up and out, find the place the first time, go through the whole procedure of getting to know people, and make a commitment to come back. But *just do it*.

In all my experience of working with addicts and their families, I have found that there is simply no substitute for this aspect of treatment. You may read all the books on the shelf and go to all the classes you can find on addiction and still not make any real progress if you don't get involved with a support group and stick with it no matter what. You may even go through extensive individual counseling and not make the kind of progress you make with a support group. I can't emphasize that enough.

### INDIVIDUAL SUPPORT

In 12-step support groups, members are encouraged to choose a sponsor—a person who is further along in recovery and who is willing to take some time to talk with you on an individual basis. Sometimes this will involve looking at the different steps and "working" them. Sometimes it will mean simply sharing your mutual experiences and looking for more productive ways to cope with problems as they arise. Going to a 12-step group without using a sponsor is rather like going without a guide to a country where you don't speak the language.

Support group meetings, however, are not places where you'll want to talk about sensitive personal information. Even though most groups insist on anonymity and confidentiality, it's not the same thing as the kind of confidentiality you are entitled to in a professional relationship with a counselor or a therapist.

Individual counseling or therapy is not a must for everyone, but it's an important adjunct for many people in recovery. You can find a good therapist by asking for referrals from a treatment center, from other support group members, or from professional associations in your area. Appendix B lists some resources to help you with this. Do be sure that your counselor or therapist is familiar with addiction and recovery.

### PSYCHIATRIC HELP

You may also need to consult with a psychiatrist for problems with depression or anxiety, or if you are feeling overwhelmed. A psychiatrist is a good resource person, too. A comprehensive psychiatric assessment with a review of your activities in recovery can be very helpful. The psychiatrist might be able to make suggestions or useful referrals. On occasion, medications are prescribed for symptoms if they are beginning to interfere with your functioning or coping skills. Seek out a psychiatrist who is familiar with addiction and recovery, preferably one who is board certified in addiction psychiatry. You can check the appendix for ways to locate a qualified psychiatrist in your area.

If you have picked up this book because you have a family member who is addicted, I urge you to get started right away with your own recovery. Let me conclude this chapter with a little story about a woman I know who has been active in Al-Anon for a number of years and is one of the happiest people I know.

Kathleen's husband was alcoholic, as was her father. Their marriage was in serious trouble, and, when it looked as if her husband would lose his job because of his drinking, she began going to Al-Anon meetings. She told the group how, one day, she had finally realized what it was all about. Her six-year-old had been playing with a toy truck, and one of the wheels had fallen off. He brought it to her, and, while she was trying to fix it, he kept reaching up to help. When she saw that she couldn't get the wheel back on with his little hand in the way, she told him to sit nearby. It wasn't long before the truck was fixed. She realized, suddenly, that this was what she had been doing for years when it came to her husband's drinking. She would ask God to help, and then get in the way because she wanted it fixed now, although she was afraid it really wasn't fixable. She learned in Al-Anon that she didn't have to fix it, that she couldn't fix it. She could sit nearby and let God work. She said, "I don't get into triangles anymore." Although it took several years, her husband eventually went to treatment and is now in recovery.

There is hope.

# 7. Recovery from Addiction

If you've decided that you have an addiction, the next question is what are you going to do about it? You've probably already tried several tactics, such as cutting down on the amount that you use, or using only on particular days (like weekends), or switching to another substance (from liquor to beer, from marijuana to alcohol). You may have gone for extended periods of time without using, but then eventually the addiction crept back in. You may be in a treatment center now, or you may have been told you will be put in a treatment center if you don't stop. Some sort of negative consequence may be hanging over your head, like a hearing for a DUI or a spouse who's left you until you get straightened out.

Whatever the reason might be, you didn't get to this point spontaneously. As the director of a treatment center often said to new admissions, "*Nobody* quits just because they wake up one day and decide they want to." Something usually has to happen to tip the balance, to push you off the fence. This is what we commonly call "hitting bottom." The question is—just how much does it take? Clinicians who work with addiction put forth a lot of effort to see that a person gets off the elevator before it hits the bottom floor.

Hitting bottom means coming to the conclusion that you are "sick and tired of being sick and tired." You are not getting the same pleasure from the substances you are using, and they are no longer eliminating uncomfortable feelings. You don't feel so good anymore when you are using, but you feel worse when you aren't. If you're addicted to alcohol, one of the depressant drugs, or an opiate, you have the additional problem of the discomfort of withdrawal whenever you decide to stop using.

Many people will stay in this situation for a long time. You can talk yourself into almost anything, and if you really feel you have no choice but to continue using, you really have to crank up the denial. It becomes very important to find some justification to keep using and to block out the painful awareness that the addiction is destroying you.

A number of circumstances can keep you stuck in this situation and prevent you from successfully getting into recovery. Some of the most common ones involve your family. We'll take a moment to look at these in more detail.

This section is for all concerned loved ones. Even though they have much at stake when it comes to the addict getting into recovery, they are also most likely to get in the way. Family members cannot help the addict get past this stage by pointing out the futility of continuing the addiction. In fact, what happens is that they become an additional reason for the addict to keep using; the person will regard the stress they are creating as a reason to continue. Many arguments between an addict and a concerned loved one are actually stereotypical games. In other words, an argument is going on at one level and a manipulation at another. Here's an example:

> John brings home a six-pack after work and pops one open in front of his wife.
>
> Mary (after a long pause and a sullen stare): "I thought you said you weren't going to drink on weeknights. You told me the other day you were getting tired of the hangovers at work."
>
> John (expletive deleted): "I've *just* gotten home and you're at it again. I've had a bad day *which* you didn't ask me about. I just need to relax."
>
> Mary: "I was just trying to help. You said . . ."
>
> John: "*Don't* tell me what I said. This is my house. If I want a beer I'll drink it."

Mary: "There's no need to shout at me."

John: "There you go again. If you'd just act like a wife instead of a warden . . ."

Mary: "I *am* your wife and I *care* about you! That's the only reason I brought it up. I thought you said you were going to cut down."

John (finishing the beer, grabbing his keys and the rest of the six-pack, and heading for the door): "I'm going out for a while. I just can't relax around here."

John has just manipulated the situation so that he has a new excuse to drink. But Mary has also been engaging in manipulation. She is trying to mold John into the person she wants him to be, and what's happened is that the interaction between the two is no longer about drinking but about who is going to call the shots in John's life.

We know that there are some particular personality changes that take place while addiction is developing, and a tendency to resist any input from others is one of them. Newcomers at AA meetings are sometimes told (gently), "You need to take the cotton out of your ears and put it in your mouth." Part of the denial system is to maintain control at all times over any negative input, and a good way to do this is to take the offense so that any such input can be neutralized.

As an addict, you need to recognize that another way your family can interefere with your getting off the fence is through well-meaning "help." You probably have some-one on whom you have come to rely when there is trouble. As we saw in chapter 5, this person is called an enabler— someone who serves as a buffer between you and negative consequences. People become enablers for a number of rea-sons, but these aren't relevant to you at this point. What's important is that you realize that the enablers in your life may unwittingly, and with the best intentions, undermine your motivation to take the difficult first steps toward recovery.

You do have a choice about the way you respond to en-abling: you can allow it to continue, or you can choose to take responsibility for the consequences of your addiction. Recovery has a lot to do with beginning to take back personal responsibility for your actions and choices. Choosing to recover means change, and this will be threatening to your loved ones. But you are the only one who can do it. If you recognize this behavior, you need to begin to gently change direction. Here's an example:

> John: "The boss told me today that if I don't go to the evening alcohol treatment program I'm going to lose my job. Mary, I'm going to have to do this. I need to do this."
>
> Mary: "What's that—the evening program?"
>
> John: "It's groups on Mondays, Tuesdays, and Thursdays. Three hours a night. And on the other nights I have to go to meetings and get an attendance slip signed."
>
> Mary: "That's ridiculous! They can't expect you to be gone every night of the week."
>
> John: "They do."
>
> Mary: "Remember last summer when you stopped drinking for over a month? Can't you just do that?"
>
> John: "It's not that simple. I have to do this or I'll lose my job."
>
> Mary: "You've hated this job anyway. Look. You can just quit like you did last year, and let me help you. If you want to drink, we'll just talk about it."
>
> John: "Mary, I know you mean well. But I have to do this. I don't want to be gone every evening either. But you have to understand. I'm an alcoholic. I realize that now."
>
> Mary: "You're a heavy drinker—you're not an . . ."
>
> John: "I'm going to do this."

John has reached the point where he realizes that he is going to have to do something about his addiction to alcohol. And this is threatening to Mary. It is more comfortable for her to try to maintain control, even though this hasn't worked in the past. It will also be very uncomfortable for John to continue to work on his addiction under these conditions, but at this point he has to put up with some conflict at home, for now, in order to get better.

So, hitting bottom is the realization that you are stuck between a rock and a hard place and that recovery is the only realistic way out. Believing that recovery is possible at this point is another matter. Many addicts and alcoholics don't try because they believe, deep down, that recovery will be a failure, too, as much else in their lives has been. After many negative consequences—broken relationships, lost jobs, legal problems—it can be difficult to believe that recovery is possible. It may help to know then that most people who have succeeded in recovery have been at exactly the same point, hopeless and helpless.

### Intervention and Court-Mandated Treatment

What if someone you care deeply about is headed in a rapid downward spiral and seems not to realize that there is a serious problem? You might be afraid that the addiction will lead to incarceration or death, as it often does, and you want to *do* something. This is a different situation from that of a family member who is emotionally invested in controlling the addict, like Mary in the vignettes. This feeling arises out of your knowledge of the severe danger your loved one is in and out of a sense of caring and concern. You see your loved one running full speed ahead toward a cliff, and you want to try to prevent disaster.

The first thing you should do is to make a commitment to go to 12-step meetings for the family members of addicts and alcoholics (Al-Anon, Narc-Anon and others). Pick out a convenient meeting, and go, today if possible. There is probably a listing in your phone book for AA; they will have the information you need. Two other strategies—intervention and court-ordered treatment—are both tricky from an emotional and relational standpoint. You not only need the support and encouragement you will get from these meetings, but you will also have to look at how your loved one's addiction has affected your coping skills and your overall mental health.

The term "intervention" indicates a procedure used by addiction professionals; it is designed to bring the addict rapidly to a point where treatment is accepted. It is somewhat controversial and if not properly conceived and carried out can be quite dangerous. In short, don't try this on your own.

Intervention is generally intiated by a family member, an employer, or a colleague. It involves taking extensive history from the people who know the addict best and who are most concerned about his or her situation. A list is made of the specific negative consequences that have occurred as a result of the addiction. A plan for getting the addict into a comprehensive treatment program is also devised and set out in advance. The addict is summoned to the intervention, usually not suspecting that family members and others are going to be present. The professional who is orchestrating the intervention will then lead the group through a presentation of the various negative consequences of the addiction, the intention being to break down denial and resistance to treatment. The addict is then presented with a choice between the previously laid-out treatment plan and some type of negative consequence, such as being fired or losing an important relationship.

Intervention is very dangerous emotionally for the addict as well as for the family. It should be carried out only by addiction professionals who are licensed and experienced in this specific technique. It should be done in a supportive manner, and, before the intervention, the confronters (family members, friends, coworkers) should be given ample opportunity to work out their anger at the addict's behavior. The purpose of the session is not to give the participants an opportunity to ventilate anger but to use a form of emotional manipulation to help the addict "hit bottom" before it's too late.

Court-mandated treatment is available in some states through a commitment procedure. Since it means temporarily suspending the addict's civil rights, it involves due process and is carried out through the court. Although the laws in each state vary, they are all based on the premise that the addict is not able to make rational choices about the addiction. A family member or some other interested party can make an application to the court for a hearing and will be required to testify as to the reason for the request. The addict is given a chance to refute any testimony given and is represented by an attorney. If the court decides that it is in the best interest of the addict to go to a treatment center, an order is written by the judge, and the addict has to go. The treatment facility must also be involved in this decision and must be willing to accept the addict as a patient. Many state-run and some private facilities will accept involuntary patients.

Family members are often hesitant to take the step of using an involuntary court commitment. One major reason is a fear that their loved one will never forgive them. Also, there may be subtle and not-so-subtle threats made by the addict if the possiblity of involuntary commitment arises. It is best to consult with a professional on this matter.

If the recommendation is made to proceed with commitment, family members should remember that addiction is a progressive and extremely destructive disease that may be fatal. Short of recovery, nothing good is going to come of the situation. The most loving thing they can do is to get the addict into circumstances where it is possible for recovery to occur, and many addicts who are court-ordered to treatment by family members eventually come to see this.

Another concern that family members frequently express about court-ordered commitment comes from the erroneous belief that the addict has to admit the problem and ask for help *before* entering treatment, so that there would be no use in committing someone to involuntary treatment. Although it is correct that at some point an addict has to take personal responsibility for recovery, it is also true that every addict—even someone in deep denial—has some degree of ambivalence about the addiction. The addict may desperately want to get rid of the addiction but not believe that it is possible to recover, or may be fearful of giving up the option of getting high because of painful inner conflicts or past trauma. In a treatment setting, even if the person arrives involuntarily, these issues can be addressed. Long-term outcomes for addicts who come to treatment voluntarily and for those who are intially court-ordered are actually about the same.

### What Exactly Is "Recovery"?

Recovery is the term used to describe the process of bringing the addiction into remission. Remember that there is no cure for this problem. Once the brain has become addicted, it stays that way. However, even though the disease of addiction remains, it can be successfully managed. It is possible to stop using the addictive substance and to be happy that you did.

Recovery proceeds in stages. The first involves coming to the point where the choice is made to stop using and to change. People usually have a lot of mixed feelings at this stage: fear of coping without the drugs or alcohol, worry that staying abstinent is not possible, a longing for the initial benefits of the substance, shame or guilt about negative consequences, anger at loved ones who coerced treatment.

Some physical consequences of the addiction are likely, depending on what drug was used, and there might be symptoms of withdrawal to contend with. Professional help is very important at this point. You need a physical check-up, and you may need detoxification. Counseling helps you deal with fears and with mixed emotions. Many alcohol and drug counselors are also recovering from addiction and can relate very personally to what you are going through.

A decision has to be made as to whether you need residential treatment—for example, in a hospital setting—or outpatient treatment. In years past, twenty-one- or twenty-eight-day inpatient programs were standard. In recent years, there has been a push towards developing outpatient options, much of it coming from insurance companies that limit reimbursement for inpatient programs.

Limited social support, physical problems, complicated addictions, and the presence of other psychiatric disorders like depression or anxiety are indicators of the need for inpatient treatment. A person's failure to remain abstinent in an outpatient program also suggests the need for residential treatment.

The bottom line is that making progress in recovery is time-consuming. If it takes a month in a hospital setting, or three months, that's what it takes. Some people are able to successfully utilize outpatient programs, but many are not. It's important to remember that this is a serious and long-term kind of problem, no matter what the constraints may be on insurance coverage. Public sector programs, such as those run by mental health centers or state hospitals, sometimes provide for a longer stay at a reduced cost, since they are subsidized by government funds.

### Alcohol and Drug Treatment Programs

Whether inpatient or outpatient, most treatment programs have certain basic features. First, medical attention and support are provided around the initial crisis that brought you to treatment. Psychiatric consultation may also be requested.

Next, there is individual assessment and counseling. You will be expected to participate in classes about addiction and in groups where you learn to talk about your feelings with the aid of a trained counselor.

Groups are particularly valuable for people with addictions. In this kind of setting, you are able to see problems in other group members that you might not be able to see in yourself. You also experience support and come to see that you are not alone, which is helpful because addictions are very isolating.

Treatment centers usually have strict rules, and they are enforced. You will, of course, be expected not to use drugs or drink while you are there. You will be advised not to get into intimate relationships with other patients. You might be told that you cannot have novels or magazines to read, and there might be a dress code. Such rules help you maintain your focus on recovery and not get sidetracked. Denial and the cravings associated with early recovery can be subtle and easily undermine treatment.

Treatment programs should offer help for the family as well. Conferences with your family and the counselor are usually included, and the family is encouraged to come to educational meetings about addiction as well as to a support group. Family members are encouraged to begin attending Al-Anon or similar programs.

Most treatment programs provide an introduction to 12-step recovery, and include attendance at Alcoholics Anonymous or Narcotics Anonymous meetings. Cognitive-behavioral therapy may also be offered. This technique teaches you to examine your thoughts and feelings and to make better choices. Relapse prevention strategies are taught as well.

### Medications Used in Addiction Treatment

A variety of medications are used to treat addiction. Initially, you may be placed on a detoxification protocol. This will vary according to the drug you are using, the degree of withdrawal, and what your medical situation is. Since depression and anxiety often linger for several months after detoxification and may interfere with sobriety, you may be placed on a medication to help correct this problem. Some commonly used in treatment centers for this purpose are fluoxetine (Prozac), imipramine (Tofranil), and valproate (Depakote). These medications have been shown to help stabilize mood in the early stages of recovery, and they are not addictive. After six months to a year, they can often be withdrawn.

Disulfiram (Antabuse) is used to prevent relapse in alcoholics. When disulfiram is in the system, it causes a violently ill reaction if someone drinks. It works best for alcoholics who drink in a binge fashion and who have trouble abstaining. It must be taken daily, and its use should be closely supervised by a physician. Since it can cause severe reactions when alcohol is ingested, certain over-the-counter drugs, mouthwashes containing alcohol, and foods containing alcohol must be avoided. Giving Antabuse to people without telling them (this has been done by some misguided family members) is highly dangerous and unethical.

Naltrexone (Trexan or Revia) blocks opiate receptors. It is used in the treatment of alcoholics as well as opiate addicts. The regular use of naltrexone has been shown to reduce the frequency and severity of relapses in alcoholics. It blocks the pleasurable sensation associated with the use of opiates and is therefore thought to be useful for recovering opiate addicts. It may also reduce the strength of cravings. It must be taken daily. Longer-acting preparations are being developed.

If you have an addiction to heroin or other opiates, you may be placed on methadone maintenance. The doctor figures out the dose of methadone you need to avoid symptoms of opiate withdrawal, and this is given two or three times a week in a controlled outpatient clinic. Well-run methadone clinics also offer ongoing counseling and therapy, and some people are able eventually to achieve full abstinence through these programs. Longer-acting drugs similar to methadone and other variations of the methadone molecule are being introduced that allow for more flexibility in the clinic routines where methadone maintenance programs are being carried out.

So far there is no drug available that can correct the emotional, psychological, and spiritual problems associated with addiction. I don't think there ever will be. Drug therapy that can help reduce relapses and keep people focused on treatment issues is useful, and should be considered as part of your treatment plan. After initial detoxification, however, many people do well without any additional medication. The use of medication in recovery is an individual decision to be made by you and your doctor.

What about sleep? In the first few weeks of treatment consider yourself lucky if you sleep, especially if you are coming off alcohol, depressants, marijuana, or opiates. If you are coming off cocaine or amphetamines you might sleep all the time at first but later have trouble getting to sleep.

Addictive drugs tend to disrupt the natural process of sleep. If we do a brain wave recording while a person is sleeping, we can see that brain waves go through several distinct stages over and over again throughout the course of the night: light sleep, dreaming sleep, and deep sleep, with the cycle then repeating itself. These cycles each last about ninety minutes. Alcohol and depressants suppress the dreaming part of sleep. Other drugs deplete the stores of chemicals that are needed to generate sleep cycles, and it takes time for these to build back up.

The bad news about this is that your doctor is probably not going to give you anything to make you sleep. Sometimes nonmood-altering antidepressants such as trazodone (Desyrel) are used at night and help with sedation, especially if there is a problem with depression or anxiety. But you might just be told to grin and bear it. The good news is that no one ever died from sleep deprivation at a treatment center, and it *will* get better with time. A peaceful night's sleep without chemicals is one of the blessings of recovery.

### Early Recovery

When you are discharged from the treatment center, you are still not well. You will be encouraged to attend 12-step meetings, often with the instruction to attend "ninety meetings in ninety days." When you step out the door of the treatment center, you step into early recovery.

Early recovery lasts about two years. Your main task at this point is to remain abstinent. At times this might be all that you can focus on, especially for the first few months. Your 12-step meetings and support from other group members is crucial at this point. You are not likely to be able to do this alone.

Here are some sayings from Alcoholics Anonymous that you'll probably find useful in getting through these first few months:

"One day at a time." You don't have to promise that you will never use or drink again. You don't have that much control over the future. But you can do it for twenty-four hours.

"Keep it simple." Just do the things that you need to do. Don't complicate your life, and don't analyze things to death. Go to meetings, read your Big Book (*Alcoholics Anonymous*), talk to your sponsor. Just for today don't drink or use.

"First things first." Rome wasn't built in a day. The problems you might have with your job, your family, or your finances are not going to get solved right away. Jumping back into work or into conflicted relationships too early is a common cause of relapse. Keep sobriety and recovery your first priority.

"This, too, shall pass." You are not accustomed to feelings. You have been avoiding unpleasant sensations for so long that you may be surprised by feelings of anger, sadness, frustration, or grief. Learning how to deal with emotions is like building up muscle tone—you have to go easy at first, then gradually develop more strength. Your support group will help. And the feelings will pass. Try to remember that the better able you are to tolerate the bad feelings, the more you will be able to experience joy and contentment.

"Stay in today." It's easy to get caught up in worrying

about the future or regretting the past. As some have put it, "Yesterday is a cancelled check, and tomorrow is a promissory note. Today is the only cash I have." Keep your focus on what you have to do today, and do it as well as you can. It gets better.

### Dealing with Relapse

Many people relapse during the first year of recovery. The single most common reason I hear for people being readmitted to treatment is that they stopped going to meetings and stopped doing the things they were taught to do in treatment. Remember that addiction is never cured. It only goes into remission. And it probably doesn't get better while it's in remission—in fact, some people believe that it gets worse.

Relapse doesn't start with using again. It starts a long time before you pick the addiction back up, in the form of attitudes and feelings. That is why ongoing support is so important. Outcome studies done on people who have completed treatment clearly show that the people who do best are the ones who continue to attend meetings and participate in recommended follow-up.

Remember, too, not to throw the baby out with the bath water. If you slip and use again, don't consider your recovery to be over. Go back to your meetings and get back in touch with your counselor or doctor. Do something. There are important reasons why you slipped and if you are going to be successful you have to understand them.

It may be that you need some additional treatment, such as counseling or psychotherapy, or that you need medication. It may be that you have family problems that have not yet been addressed. Whatever it is, it's fixable as long as you are willing to deal with it. In fact, it's not uncommon for some people to go through treatment several times before getting it right.

## Middle Recovery

The middle phase of recovery lasts from about the third year to the tenth year or beyond. At this point, you are fairly secure with abstinence and with your recovery program. You may begin working on longer-term problems that have stayed on the back burner during the first couple of years. Many people return to school, or find a better job. Now that life is less chaotic, there is time for other pursuits and new relationships. Some people experience a revived interest in religion or in civic activities.

You might find, though, that you are still struggling with feelings of depression or anxiety and that you are not experiencing the joy and contentment you expected. Longer-term issues might need to be addressed. Many people who develop addiction come from dysfunctional families and may have experienced abuse and neglect as children. It's also very common for other psychiatric problems such as clinical depression or anxiety disorders to be present.

A common misconception in the recovering community is that working on your program alone should make you happy. This just isn't so for a lot of people. You may be doing everything right and still be struggling. If you're not yet feeling good at this stage you should seek evaluation from a psychiatrist or psychologist who understands addiction. Relapse is still possible—it's always possible—and there is effective treatment available if you ask for it.

## Late Recovery

In the later stages of recovery, some people begin to loosen their attachment to 12-step programs and become emotionally invested in other relationships and pursuits. But many people remain quite active in their meetings, serving as sponsors for newcomers and keeping the meetings going. Without these "old-timers" the 12-step programs would cease to exist.

The risk of relapse continues. Many of those who remain active in 12-step groups maintain that they would relapse if they stopped going. I certainly can't argue with that. Problems with depression, loss, and the stresses of aging are common. The ongoing support of the 12-step meetings is very helpful. Without it, some people feel that their thinking and attitudes begin to regress to the "stinking thinking" that characterized the addiction.

Outcome studies have shown that people who continue to be active in recovery programs show remarkable growth over the long term. Gradual development of the personality occurs, along with resolution of old conflicts. Relationships improve, and the damage caused by the addiction can be repaired.

There are those, however, who seem to stall out in recovery. They may continue to attend meetings, and they may remain abstinent, but personal growth stops. These people are at increased risk for later relapse, and may benefit from long-term psychotherapy to address personality issues.

### What Is Alcoholics Anonymous?

During the early decades of the twentieth century, a man named Bill Wilson, a talented entrepreneur and businessman, was sinking deeper into addiction to alcohol. He tried everything available at that time to give it up but would always eventually return to drinking, as his career and home life deteriorated. He sought opinions about his drinking problem from experts and found that there were no satisfactory answers.

He eventually encountered a friend and old drinking buddy who was sober, happy, and apparently doing well. What his friend had discovered was that by giving his "struggle over to God" and by "taking it one day at a time" he was able to stay sober; his life had turned around, and he was happier than he had ever been. Bill Wilson took the same steps.

Recognizing that he had to be of service to others in order to stay sober, he began to spread the word by calling on alcoholics who were willing to listen—those in hospital wards or on the streets—and simply relating his experiences and offering to listen. By 1935, the organization Alcoholics Anonymous was born. Today there are tens of millions of members worldwide. The 12 steps of Alcoholics Anonymous have been adopted and utilized by people with all types of addictions and behavior problems; groups include Overeaters Anonymous, Gamblers Anonymous, Narcotics Anonymous, and Codependents Anonymous.

The basic premise of 12-step recovery is a spiritual one. It is based on the conviction that addiction involves spiritual bankruptcy characterized mainly by "self-will run riot." Recovery begins by admitting that the addiction is out of your control and that your life is out of control. This is the first step, and it is an admission of hopelessness. What happens next is best decribed in the Big Book in chapter 2, "There Is a Solution." The chapter tells of a man's trip to Europe to consult with Dr. Carl Jung, a noted psychoanalyst, about his alcoholism:

> Some of our alcoholic readers may think they can do without spiritual help. Let us tell you the rest of the conversation our friend had with his doctor.
>
> The doctor said: "You have the mind of a chronic alcoholic. I have never seen one single case recover, where that state of mind existed to the extent that it does in you." Our friend felt as though the gates of hell had closed in on him with a clang.
>
> He said to the doctor, "Is there no exception?"
>
> "Yes," replied the doctor, "there is. Exceptions to cases such as yours have been occurring since early times. Here and there, once in a while, alcoholics have had what are called vital spiritual experiences. To me these occurrences are phenomena. They appear to be in the nature of huge emotional displacements and rearrangements. Ideas, emotions, and attitudes which were

once the guiding forces of the lives of these men are suddenly cast to one side, and a completely new set of conceptions and motives begins to dominate them. In fact, I have been trying to produce some such emotional rearrangement within you. With many individuals the methods which I employed are successful, but I have never been successful with an alcoholic of your description."

Upon hearing this, our friend was somewhat relieved, for he reflected that, after all, he was a good church member. This hope, however, was destroyed by the doctor's telling him that while his religious convictions were very good, in his case they did not spell the necessary spiritual experience.

Here was the terrible dilemma in which our friend found himself when he had the extraordinary experience, which as we have already told you, made him a free man.

We, in our turn, sought the same escape with all the desperation of drowning men. What seemed at first a flimsy reed has proved to be the loving and powerful hand of God. A new life has been given us or, if you prefer, "a design for living" that really works.

The original members of Alcoholics Anonymous were quick to point out that this was not a religious program, even though there is an emphasis on God. Instead they stressed the importance of personal spirituality in the process of recovery. They recognized that many alcoholics had problems with the concept of God, and the final version of the book *Alcoholics Anonymous* contained the additional words "*as we understood Him*" when God was mentioned in the 12 steps. A belief in God is not necessary in order to begin recovering through a 12-step program, but a "spiritual awakening" is part of a successful 12-step recovery. Recovering alcoholics and addicts in 12-step programs often express gratitude, saying that when the addiction knocked them to their knees was when they found God.

Many people find that their addiction goes into remission

following a spiritual conversion. Church-based addiction programs emphasize spiritual growth and religious maturity. The basic concept of recovery here is not very different from Alcoholics Anonymous and the other 12-step programs, but these approaches include a doctrinal aspect specific to a religion.

People who have a spiritual conversion, stop drinking or using drugs, and start attending church without professional help or AA attendance sometimes run into snags. In some churches a stigma is associated with addiction that makes it difficult to talk honestly about day-to-day problems. Some churches have legalistic doctrines, and the addict is tempted to adopt a set of rules that substitutes for actual recovery. Long-term abstinence in this situation can be difficult, and relapse can damage the addict's faith. There are addiction and mental health professionals who can work effectively with religious beliefs, and most religious doctrines dovetail nicely with the principles of 12-step recovery. For example, church attendance and Bible study along with regular 12-step meetings is a good combination. As one AA member put it, "I go to church to save my soul. I go to AA meetings to save my behind." Crudely put, maybe, but useful advice.

But what if you are agnostic or atheistic? A number of solutions are available. The reference to "a power greater than ourselves" in step 2 offers the possibility of accepting a "higher power"—not necessarily God—to help with recovery. Sometimes people begin with just the awareness that the addiction is beyond their personal power, and they rely on the support of the group as a higher power.

One woman, early in recovery, was told by her AA sponsor that she needed to pray if she was to have another sober day. She had been raised Catholic but had turned away from the church in her teens. She started out not believing in God, but she knew she had no option other than to try and do what her AA sponsor told her to do. She began praying to "Howard"—and got sober for the first time in her adult life. She later explained that she prayed to Howard because of how she had first heard the Lord's Prayer as a child: "Our father, which art in heaven, *Howard* be thy name . . ." Another woman in treatment had a small rubber ball that she kept with her at all times. She explained that this was her higher power. She did not believe in God, but she had started out on the road to recovery.

Of course, the "God thing" remains problematic. Atheists and agnostics may object to the emphasis on God in 12-step recovery (contrary to popular belief, the Big Book unapologetically refers to "God" again and again, and not just to the concept of a "higher power"). Conservative religious people sometimes object to the lack of emphasis on doctrine. Some people have characterized AA as a type of cult religion that comes to substitute for the original addiction.

Various research approaches have attempted to define and analyze what the effective factors are in 12-step recovery. An increase in a sense of self-efficacy, renewed connection with others in the context of the group, and the repair of attitudes and relationships are some which have been studied. But many recovering people and addiction professionals consider the activity of a loving God in the recovering person's life to be a real and effective factor in successful recovery. A lot of the addicts I've seen in my practice who are unable to stay sober for more than a few weeks or months have trouble with the "God thing," and they use their discomfort with the spiritual aspects of AA to avoid getting involved. Sometimes this is a symptom of denial, sometimes it comes from deep-seated hurts and disappointments that have occurred in their lives, and sometimes it indicates an unwillingness to admit that there is something going on with them that they cannot control.

Does this mean that being atheistic or agnostic makes it impossible to get sober and bring the addiction into remission? No. The concepts within the 12 steps can be adapted, and behaviors changed through strategies like cognitive-behavioral or reality therapy—approaches that encourage you to look at your behaviors, your basic assumptions, and the consequences of your actions, and begin to make better choices. Rational recovery is a program available in some urban areas which provides group support within a nonspiritual context. If you are atheistic or agnostic these programs may work for you. But if you have struggled with staying clean, and nothing seems to be working, you may need to reflect carefully on the spiritual aspect of your life. A chapter in *Alcoholics Anonymous* entitled "We Agnostics" is worth reading.

Moderation management is another strategy for the treatment of alcohol abuse that has a following, but it is viewed with skepticism by many addiction professionals, and I am among them. The idea behind moderation management is that alcoholics can learn to drink socially if given enough support and input. The problem I have with this approach is that it flies in the face of what we know scientifically about addiction and the changes that occur in the brain. People who have been successful in moderation management programs may be people who were abusing alcohol, but did not develop actual addiction.

Most addiction treatment centers introduce patients to the concepts of 12-step recovery and include AA or NA meetings in their schedules. But anyone can go to an AA meeting. According to the AA preamble, "the only requirement for membership is a desire to stop drinking." Closed meetings are for alcoholics or addicts only. Open meetings, which often feature a speaker, are open to family members or other interested individuals as well.

Anonymity, or confidentiality, is stressed in 12-step groups. The opening announcements often include this directive: "Who you see here, what you hear here, when you leave here, let it stay here." Only first names are used, and people are encouraged to drop the usual social barriers; a lawyer might be sitting next to a pipe fitter who is sitting next to a society matron, and so on.

Several varieties of 12-step meetings exist: speaker meetings, when one or two members relate their stories, discussion meetings, which involve the entire group and usually center on a topic, and step study and Big Book meetings, where detailed study of the 12 steps and other related material is undertaken.

These are not "group therapy" sessions. Highly personal issues are generally not discussed, and "cross talk"—one member addressing another—is frowned upon. Members are encouraged to talk about their own experiences with recovery and share their "experience, strength and hope."

A good 12-step meeting has a warm and accepting atmosphere. Most addicts have had problems with social anxiety, and the fear of being confronted or shamed keeps many people away from these meetings. Recovering people know this, and will usually go out of their way to welcome newcomers and help them feel comfortable.

When you start out in 12-step recovery, it is suggested that you choose someone as a sponsor. A sponsor is another person in recovery who helps with working the steps and dealing with more personal problems on a one-to-one basis. A sponsor should be someone of the same sex who has had several years of good recovery. At first, you can request telephone numbers of people available as temporary sponsors or phone contacts and take time to get to know the group before choosing a sponsor.

When you're starting out in 12-step recovery, it's also a good idea to check out a number of different meetings. Meetings have different atmospheres and personalities; it's not a "one fits all" situation. Go several times to a meeting before you decide whether or not you like it. You might hit one on a bad night or a good night. You want to be familiar with what's average for that meeting. Some people attend different meetings in different locations on different nights. That way they have a chance to hear a variety of points of view. If you find a group that you like you can choose it as your "home group."

**The Twelve Steps of Alcoholics Anonymous**

1. We admitted we were powerless over alcohol—that our lives had become unmanageable.

2. Came to believe that a power greater than ourselves could restore us to sanity.

3. Made a decision to turn our will and our lives over to the care of God *as we understood Him.*

4. Made a searching and fearless moral inventory of ourselves.

5. Admitted to God, to ourselves, and to another human being the exact nature of our wrongs.

6. Were entirely ready to have God remove all these defects of character.

7. Humbly asked Him to remove our shortcomings.

8. Made a list of all persons we had harmed, and became willing to make amends to them all.

9. Made direct amends to such people wherever possible, except when to do so would injure them or others.

10. Continued to take personal inventory and when we were wrong promptly admitted it.

11. Sought through prayer and meditation to improve our conscious contact with God *as we understood Him*, praying only for knowledge of His will for us and the power to carry that out.

12. Having had a spiritual awakening as the result of these steps, we tried to carry this message to alcoholics, and to practice these principles in all our affairs.

From: *Alcoholics Anonymous*, 3rd Edition, 1976
Alcoholics Anonymous World Services, Inc.
New York, New York

The 12 steps describe the process that the original members of Alcoholics Anonymous went through in their search for sobriety. There is nothing magical about them. The first 3 steps relate what happens when an addict finally hits bottom and realizes that there is really no hope that life can continue the way it has been going. Combined with that sense of hopelessness and powerlessness, however, is the realization

that it is possible to recover. Deciding to put faith and trust
in the process and be open to help completes the first 3 steps.
It is not critical at this point that you make any final decisions
about who God is, or even that there is a God. All that is
necessary is that you look around and see that there are other
people who are sober and happy and then to become open-
minded and willing to do the things they did to get sober.

Steps 4 through 9 are reparative. In the process of working
these steps you take an honest look at your life and personality and become ready to make changes. This doesn't happen
overnight. You can take as long as you need to complete
these steps. And you can go back and do them over if you
like. There is no correct time frame. You don't want to put
them off, but there's no advantage in rushing them either.
Included in these steps is a process of making amends to
people you may have harmed as the result of your addiction
or your behaviors. Although this can be very difficult, it is
remarkably helpful. You might not be able to reconcile some
relationships, but you can get a sense of peace about them.

Steps 10 through 12 are concerned with maintenance. These
involve an ongoing process of examining and taking responsibility for your behavior and a continuation of growth, spiritually and emotionally. Service to others, especially to other
suffering alcoholics and addicts, is an important part of maintaining your sobriety.

We have covered a lot of ground in this discussion of
recovery. If you are reading this because you have a problem
with addiction, don't feel overwhelmed. People take these
steps every day, and many recovering people are out there
to help you along the way. The first thing you can do is talk
to someone. Alcoholics Anonymous is listed in most phone
books at the very beginning under AA. Even if your problem
is drugs or a behavioral addiction like gambling, the person
on the other end of the line will help you get started.

# 8. Dual Diagnosis

People with addictions often have other psychiatric problems. This was documented in a 1970s survey known as the Epidemiological Catchment Area (ECA) study, in which households were polled in several geographical areas. Complete diagnostic surveys were done, and the study generated an enormous amount of statistical data that has been useful in our understanding of many different mental health problems.

We know that addictions often start with a person's desire to alter his or her mood with a substance. In uncomplicated situations, such an urge might indicate fairly minor problems, such as the shyness and awkwardness of adolescence. But often there is more serious trouble regarding emotions and mental functioning.

The ECA study showed that problems like major depression, anxiety disorders, or schizophrenia frequently coexist with addiction and that the chance of having one increases for those who have another. In other words, addiction increases the risk that other mental health problems will develop and the presence of other mental health problems increases the risk that addiction will develop.

The treatment of people with serious mental illness and addiction became a problem because of the way mental health delivery systems were set up. Starting at the federal level and going on down to state and local levels, the funding and regulation of alcohol and drug treatment programs and of mental health treatment programs have been controlled by separate agencies. As a result, professionals have clustered on one side or the other. Some people who specialize in treating addiction have little experience with other mental health problems, and the reverse is also true.

The result of this split is that people who have both types of problems sometimes fall through the cracks of the system.

In the not-too-distant past, it was common for someone to seek treatment at an alcohol and drug facility only to be sent away because of mental health problems. When the same person went to a mental health facility, treatment there was considered "inappropriate" because of the addiction problem.

Dual diagnosis programs in which both conditions are given equal emphasis have been developed over the past decade or so to address this problem. Both conditions must be treated vigorously, and specialized follow-up is sometimes included. Dual Recovery Anonymous consists of 12-step groups involved in recovery from both addiction and severe mental illness. And many facilities also offer long-term therapy groups that work with patients at any level of recovery, with the aim of keeping people engaged in the treatment process so that gradual progress can be made.

Virtually any psychiatric disorder can coexist with addiction. And addiction itself often leads to symptoms of depression and anxiety as a result of the effects of the substances and of the destructive consequences of the addiction.

We can classify these coexisting disorders into three categories: substance-induced disorders, psychiatrically complicated addiction, and serious persistent mental illness and addiction.

Those to whom the first two categories apply can usually be dealt with in traditional alcohol and drug treatment settings through psychiatric consultation and minor modifications in the treatment program. But the third category includes disorders that result in significant impairment in functioning and require a specialized approach if the treatment of both conditions is to be effective.

### Substance-Induced Disorders

These conditions or symptoms are caused by the substance being abused and would not be present otherwise. They usually clear over time with abstinence.

Depression is common in people who are addicted. The condition often results from the many negative consequences of the addiction and the sense of hopelessness it engenders. But certain drugs, especially alcohol, cocaine, and amphetamines, are particularly likely to produce depressive symptoms.

Excessive use of alcohol can lead to a condition known as alcoholic hallucinosis, in which people hear derisive voices talking to them. The condition sometimes remits with long-term abstinence but may require treatment with antipsychotic medication. It is sometimes misdiagnosed as schizophrenia.

Heavy use of the hallucinogens, PCP, or amphetamines can cause psychosis that is indistinguishable from schizophrenia. In most cases the condition will resolve with treatment, but it sometimes becomes chronic, especially following heavy PCP use.

Anxiety and panic attacks are often seen in people who abuse alcohol, sedatives, or marijuana. Symptoms of chronic withdrawal from alcohol and sedatives may be mistakenly thought to constitute an anxiety disorder. The mechanism for panic attacks in chronic marijuana users is unknown.

Substance-induced disorders often cause diagnostic problems for clinicians. These disorders and symptoms frequently resolve within a few weeks to months of abstinence and do not necessarily constitute a second primary diagnosis. When there have been distinct episodes of symptoms before the onset of the addiction, it is easier to rule out a substance-induced disorder. Otherwise, the passage of time usually clears up any questions about whether ongoing treatment for a second diagnosis is actually needed.

## Psychiatrically Complicated Addiction

This category includes people who may be in a traditional alcohol and drug treatment setting but who have additional psychiatric needs, such as individuals with histories of emotional, psychological, or sexual trauma and those with mild-to-moderate depression or anxiety disorders. Such people are able to participate in traditional approaches to the treatment of their addiction but may need medication for psychiatric symptoms and additional psychotherapy.

If these conditions are not properly identified and addressed during the course of treatment, relapse often occurs soon after discharge. As these people continue in aftercare, they may still suffer from depression, anxiety, or problems coping, and they don't realize the benefits of sobriety. Often they will give up and return to the addiction as a result.

This is one reason why aftercare and follow-up are so important, especially during the first year or so of sobriety. Many difficult issues arise during that time, and it's not uncommon for additional psychiatric problems to be identified. A person who has not begun to feel better and to function more capably after three or four months of abstinence should be evaluated for the presence of a coexisting disorder by a psychiatrist or psychologist familiar with addiction.

### Serious Persistent Mental Illness and Addiction

The people who have had the most difficulty with the split between addiction and mental health treatment delivery systems are those who suffer from the major psychiatric disorders, which are chronic and cause significant functional impairment. These conditions include schizophrenia, bipolar disorder, schizoaffective disorder, major depression, and certain personality disorders. All are associated with an increased incidence of addiction. Over the last decade there has been a push toward the development of specialized dual diagnosis programming to help meet the needs of people with these conditions.

Let's look briefly at each of these disorders and at how traditional alcohol and drug treatment approaches can be modified to enhance the chances of successful recovery for those who have them.

### Schizophrenia

Schizophrenia is a disorder of brain functioning that results in a characteristic set of symptoms. We still do not fully understand what causes schizophrenia, but there is good evidence that there are several distinct subtypes with different causes and courses. Some cases appear to be genetically based; others seem to arise from a disruption in the development of the brain, a condition that remains dormant until the person reaches a certain age.

Contrary to popular belief, no evidence exists that drug abuse causes schizophrenia. With the exception of PCP-induced psychosis and alcoholic hallucinosis, most psychotic conditions induced by drugs will readily clear with abstinence and do not become chronic. However, individuals who are biologically predisposed to develop schizophrenia can, by abusing drugs, bring about the onset of active symptoms.

The term "schizophrenia" does not mean "split personality"; it literally means "split mind," but the word is used to describe the disorganization of thinking and emotions that characterizes this disorder, not the splitting into several distinct personalities that is is seen with multiple personalities.

Roughly 1 percent of the population suffers from schizophrenia, and many of these people have significant impairment in their overall functioning. Symptoms generally appear in the late teens or early twenties, although some cases begin during childhood or later in life. Subtle childhood problems with tasks such as learning to socialize may be identified retrospectively in people who later developed schizophrenia. Psychotic symptoms such as hallucinations and delusions are seen during active phases of the disorder. In periods of remission, many people still have significant residual symptoms such as a blunting of emotional responsiveness or a decrease in the acuity of their thinking.

Disordered thinking and ability to reason are characteristic of schizophrenia. As a result, many people with schizophrenia have impaired judgment, especially in social situations. It's common for people with schizophrenia to experiment with drugs and alcohol in an effort to fit in socially, as it is for them to abuse illicit drugs in order to self-medicate ongoing symptoms or to reduce uncomfortable side effects of medication.

Some people with schizophrenia also develop addiction. If there is a genetic susceptibility to alcoholism or addiction or prolonged abuse of alcohol or drugs, addictive disease can occur, which means that the person has two serious and chronic mental health problems.

People with this disorder are often uncomfortable in social situations and in groups. The technique of direct confrontation that is used in many traditional alcohol and drug programs to address denial and personality flaws is threatening to people with schizophrenia, and they may experience a worsening of the symptoms of psychosis as a result of this stress.

Some of those with schizophrenia have difficulty maintaining attention to lectures, watching videos, and completing workbook assignments because of problems with the intellectual functions of attention, concentration, and memory that accompany this disorder. A good deal of the work done in traditional alcohol and drug treatment centers involves these types of activities, and someone with schizophrenia may seem noncompliant or uninterested if the clinician does not understand the person's difficulties in completing such tasks.

A lack of insight is another problem found in those with schizophrenic disorders. It was once thought that this characteristic was of psychological origin, but there is now good evidence that it is the result of a brain dysfunction caused by the schizophrenic disorder. The person may not realize that he or she has a mental illness and is in need of treatment, a lack of understanding that is sometimes mistaken for denial by clinicians who work primarily with addictions. Applying the same methods for reducing denial in those with addiction to a person who has a schizophrenic disorder is a frustrating experience for the clinician as well as for the patient, and often leads to the patient leaving treatment.

Schizophrenia is usually managed with a combination of medications for the psychotic symptoms and supportive therapy and counseling. A case manager, someone who serves as a contact person and facilitator, can be very helpful in fostering compliance with treatment and gradual progress towards stabilization. Psychoeducation is a combination of teaching and therapy that presents in a nonthreatening manner the facts of the illness and ways in which to manage it. People with schizophrenia need to learn how to manage stress, identify symptoms, and communicate effectively with caregivers.

Schizophrenia is a chronic illness with a relapsing course, but newer medications and treatment techniques have come a long way in reducing the impairment and disability caused by it.

### Bipolar Disorder

Bipolar disorder is a biologically based psychiatric condition that can in some cases lead to significant impairment in functioning. The disorder used to be called manic-depression, a term that was somewhat misleading since the typical pattern of manic symptoms followed by depression is not always seen.

Good evidence exists that bipolar disorder is genetically transmitted. When we look at the family histories of people with the disorder, we often find that other family members have been diagnosed with it. Sometimes family members are alcoholic or have committed suicide. A history of clinical depression or schizophrenia often represents untreated bipolar disorder or a missed diagnosis in a previous generation.

The primary problem in bipolar disorder is the regulation of mood states. Under stress, the susceptible individual will have a change in mood that is out of proportion to circumstances. Manic episodes involve an abnormal elevation of mood, decreased sleep and appetite, increased activity, racing thoughts, overtalkativeness, and impaired judgment. Mild cases are termed hypomania, which means "just short of mania." Delusions of grandeur or religious delusions can occur in severe cases. Depressive episodes involve a lowering of mood, increased sleep, increased appetite or nervous overeating, lack of interest in activities, slowed thinking, and disturbed concentration. Thoughts of suicide and actual attempts are a common complication. A mixed state occurs when there are manic symptoms of overactivity, racing thoughts, and poor sleep in combination with an irritable or depressed mood.

We see a variety of patterns in bipolar disorder. In the classic pattern, episodes of mania are followed by severe depression with periods of remission in between. Some people have isolated episodes of mania with little depression; others have more episodes of depression and only a few of mania. There are people with strong family histories of bipolar disorder who have only episodes of depression. Bipolar II, a less severe condition, involves episodes of hypomania alternating with depression. Cyclothymic disorder is characterized by an even milder instability of moods and is seen in people with a family history of bipolar disorder.

Changes in mood according to season also occur in some with bipolar disorder and are thought to be a reflection of the brain's ability to sense the amount of ambient light. A worsening of depression in the winter months and the onset of manic symptoms in the spring are common. Some people experience depression only in the winter months, with no symptoms during other seasons, a condition that is called seasonal affective disorder. The use of phototherapy (exposure to strong light for about twenty minutes a day) is helpful in these cases.

In bipolar disorder, periods of remission usually occur between episodes. Rapid cycling refers to a condition in which there are frequent episodes with little remission of symptoms.

Plotting a time line and charting the onset, duration, and type of symptoms is a useful adjunct to treatment and helps the person with bipolar disorder manage the illness.

The mainstay of treatment of bipolar disorder is the use of mood-stabilizing medications that prevent the shifts toward mania or depression. The oldest of these is lithium. Lithium is a low molecular weight ion that is administered in the form of a salt—for example, with a carbonate ion. It stabilizes the membranes of nerve cells and prevents the cycles of depression and mania.

Over the past twenty years, a number of medicines that are used to treat epilepsy have been found to be useful for bipolar disorder. The same mechanism that stabilizes brain cells and prevents seizures also prevents the mood swings of bipolar disorder. Valproate (Depakote) and carbamazepine (Tegretol) are two such medications being prescribed widely by psychiatrists. Some of the newer anticonvulsants also show promise in the treatment of bipolar disorder. Other medications such as antidepressants, minor tranquilizers, and antipsychotic medications are used to manage the different phases of bipolar disorder. It is important for a person with bipolar disorder to become familiar with all prescribed medications and learn to recognize symptoms of mania or depression in an early stage so as to prevent a full-blown episode.

Bipolar disorder can vary in severity from being a minor inconvenience to involving major impairment in all areas of functioning. Proper psychiatric management and careful compliance with treatment recommendations can reduce the disability associated with this disorder. Many people with bipolar disorder lead full and productive lives.

People with bipolar disorder are at particularly high risk of developing addiction. There may be a genetic vulnerability to both disorders. Also, people with bipolar disorder often attempt to alleviate their symptoms with alcohol or drugs, especially before the illness has been properly identified. Substance abuse intensifies the symptoms of depression and anxiety over time. Judgment is impaired as the illness becomes active, and the tendency to abuse substances increases.

Some people with bipolar disorder come to enjoy feeling slightly manic. At the early stages of a manic episode, the heightened sense of well-being and increased productivity are similar to the effects produced by stimulants such as amphetamines or cocaine. People with bipolar disorder can learn to manipulate their medications to induce this feeling. However, it's very difficult to control the effect. What usually happens is that the symptoms of mania worsen and judgment becomes impaired, leading to a loss of control.

Supportive and educative therapy is important for people with bipolar disorder, and an ongoing relationship with a psychiatrist or psychologist helps reduce the frequency of episodes. In severe cases, when there is significant impairment of functioning and judgment, case management is also helpful.

### Schizoaffective Disorder

Schizoaffective disorder is a condition that has some aspects of schizophrenia and some of bipolar disorder or major depression. For example, hallucinations, delusions, and disorganized thinking might occur along with symptoms of mania, or severe depression might be accompanied by the disordered thinking typical of schizophrenia.

Treatment approaches for schizoaffective disorder involve an individualized combination of therapies. Antipsychotic medication along with a mood stabilizer is often used. Supportive psychotherapy, case management, and education are also important.

### Major Depression

Depression involves a characteristic set of symptoms but represents a diverse group of disorders. Most cases of depression are mild to moderate and short lived. As we've seen, depressive symptoms are common in addiction and are also frequently induced by alcohol or drugs. But in some cases depression is severe and prolonged and causes significant impairment in functioning. The condition can be broken down roughly into three types: reactive or situational, developmentally based, and biologically based.

Situational or reactive depression is common in alcoholics and addicts and generally clears with counseling and medication. Developmentally based depression often results from abuse or neglect in childhood or from growing up in a dysfunctional family.

Biologically based depression, or major depression, is a disorder that affects the part of the brain responsible for maintaining mood and handling stress. It can be mild, moderate, or severe. There is often a family history of major depression. In some cases a trauma has occurred in childhood, such as the loss of a parent, which is severe enough to have affected the development of the brain, leading to a vulnerability to biologically based depression.

Symptoms include a persistently depressed mood, a lack of reactivity of mood to social interaction, slowed thinking, poor appetite, intermittent or early morning awakening, poor concentration, impaired short-term memory, and morbid preoccupation. Thoughts of suicide are often present, and there is a risk of suicide attempts. Some abnormalities in endocrine functioning have been noted, such as a blunting of the responsiveness of the thyroid gland and failure of the adrenal gland to respond to the presence of a test dose of dexamethasone (a steroid). In severe cases there may be hallucinations and delusions, often with morbid or depressed content.

Major depression usually responds to treatment with medications along with psychotherapy, but sometimes depression is resistant to treatment and leads to chronic problems with concentration, mood, and self-esteem. Addicts with treatment-resistant major depression often have difficulty with recovery since they do not share the apparent benefits of abstinence with their peers. They may also be overly sensitive to confrontation and have difficulty with the middle steps of a 12-step program.

### Personality Disorders

Personality disorders are persistent patterns of behavior and coping that lead to chronic problems with maladjustment. Psychological trauma in childhood and other problems with development are thought to contribute to the development of a personality disorder. There may also be genetic factors.

Personality disorders are resistant to change. They represent a lifelong constriction in the range of available coping strategies. People with personality disorders are unaware of problems with their behavior and tend to use projection and blaming in a defensive fashion in order to avoid introspection. In this sense, people with addiction resemble those with personality disorders. There is considerable overlap in the incidence of addiction and personality disorders; the difference is that the distortions of personality caused by addiction will gradually improve with recovery. When addiction and a personality disorder are both present, adopting a lifestyle of recovery and continued growth can be very difficult.

Antisocial personality disorder is commonly complicated by addiction for several reasons. There may be a shared genetic vulnerability. Also, people with antisocial personality tend to have difficulty learning from painful experience and to take risks. Their ability to relate to other people is significantly impaired, and relationships are shallow and exploitive. People with the disorder often become involved in criminal or abusive behaviors.

The presence of antisocial personality disorder makes success in recovery unlikely. It should be noted that this situation does not constitute a dual diagnosis in the typical sense of the term. In fact, the modifications in addiction treatment that are made for people with dual diagnosis are the opposite of what a person with antisocial personality disorder needs in order to get better. Highly confrontational and structured programs such as the therapeutic community approach of the sixties or recent prison-based "boot camp" programs are more likely to be successful for a person with this disorder who is addicted.

People with paranoid, schizoid, or schizotypal personality disorders have traits that resemble symptoms of schizophrenia. They have difficulty with socialization and with self-esteem, and sometimes do poorly in traditional alcohol and drug treatment or unmodified 12-step programs. Dual diagnosis programming is often helpful for an addict with one of these personality disorders.

Narcissistic, dependent, histrionic, and compulsive personality disorders involve various neurotic traits which lead to impaired interpersonal functioning and difficulties with jobs and academic achievement, but often do not preclude successful treatment in traditional alcohol and drug programs.

Borderline personality disorder is a complex condition that resembles a number of other severe psychiatric disorders and is unique in its responsiveness to medication and therapy. It is characterized by instability in relationships, poor stress tolerance, repeated self-destructive behavior that includes suicide gestures and attempts, severe anxiety, periods of depression, and, often, brief episodes of psychosis. Eating disorders such as bulimia or compulsive overeating may be present. Substance abuse may occur in episodes or may lead to the development of addiction. It is thought that borderline personality disorder arises from a combination of genetic vulnerability to depression and early childhood trauma. A history of such trauma, especially sexual abuse, is common in people with this disorder.

Those with borderline personality disorder have deficits in their concept of self and trouble with everyday coping. They are very sensitive to rejection or abandonment. They often respond to emotional threats by projecting their negative feelings on others or splitting the world into all good or all bad. As a result, they can appear manipulative and emotionally destructive.

In a traditional alcohol and drug program they may respond to the stress of treatment by shifting their focus to perceived flaws in the staff or by becoming involved in treatment romances. If there is a history of sexual or other severe childhood abuse, people with borderline disorder may engage in repetitive self-mutilation, such as cutting themselves superficially or burning themselves with cigarettes. These acts are carried out in order to reduce uncomfortable feelings of anxiety and detachment, but are disturbing to others, particularly staff members in a treatment setting. Following stabilization and a period of treatment in a dual diagnosis program, however, many with borderine personality disorder and addiction do well in traditional alcohol and drug treatment settings and 12-step groups.

Borderline personality disorder is treated with a combination of medications to control the unstable moods and psychotherapy. Therapy may be cognitively based, especially at first, or intensive and insight-oriented. A long course of treatment, on the order of many years, is usually necessary. Many people with borderline personality disorder—unlike those with other personality disorders—do achieve a satisfactory resolution of symptoms over time, especially if there is an opportunity for a stable work or family setting for a number of years.

### Treatment of Dually Diagnosed People

People with serious persistent mental illness and addiction often lack the ego strength and coping skills necessary to put a recovery program into action. This necessitates modifications in the treatment approach.

An important principle in the management of a dually diagnosed individual is that treatment for both conditions must receive equal emphasis and attention. Ideal programming integrates mental health care with interventions for the addiction; the patient should be receiving everything needed to treat both the psychiatric condition and the addiction.

A successful dual diagnosis program is staffed by clinicians who have had training and experience in addiction treatment as well as in the treatment of chronic mental illness. A team of professionals from different disciplines meet to discuss the needs of the client and provide a spectrum of interventions.

Intensive case management has been useful in keeping people with mental illness and addiction engaged in treatment. In this model, clients are assigned to a case manager who makes frequent contact, often going into the community to visit the client's home. The case manager makes sure that the client has medical and psychiatric follow-up and is enrolled in specific programming to address both problems. The case manager does not provide therapy but does offer interpersonal contact and support that would otherwise be lacking for a person with impaired social functioning. Over time, a trusting relationship develops which allows the case manager to be more effective in helping the client make better choices about using alcohol or drugs.

Clinic-based groups that focus on addiction and mental illness are an important feature of dual diagnosis programming. These groups are led by a therapist, and combine education about substance abuse with an opportunity for structured interaction. Motivational group therapy is a nondirective approach that helps clients examine their behaviors without fearing judgment or criticism. In such a group setting people with different degrees of success with sobriety can provide useful feedback and role modeling.

Sometimes hospitalization or residential treatment is needed. Residential programs for the dually diagnosed utilize a team approach. Long-term stays are often needed so that problems with both the mental illness and the addiction can be fully addressed. If the mental illness is active at the time of admission, it may be a while before the person is able to look at the addiction. Nonetheless, interventions aimed at increasing awareness of addiction and its consequences should occur early in the course of hospitalization, in a supportive and nonthreatening manner.

People with serious mental illness often do poorly in AA or other 12-step groups. Since they are deficient in social functioning, they may act inappropriately or misinterpret the statements and behaviors of others. Occasionally the content of the 12 steps triggers religious delusions. The emphasis on abstinence from all mood-altering substances may also be misinterpreted as permission to stop taking needed medication.

Dual Recovery Anonymous groups are available in some locations. These are 12-step groups composed of people with both serious mental illness and addiction. Sometimes they are sponsored by a mental health clinic and are facilitated by a therapist. The principles in the 12 steps are used not only to deal with the addiction but also to promote acceptance of the chronic mental illness and personal responsibility for recovery from both conditions.

As treatments improve for serious persistent mental illness, people with these disorders suffer fewer residual symptoms during periods of remission and fewer side effects from medication. But there remain a large number of people with addiction and mental illness who are alienated from the system of care. Many of them are homeless and destitute. Assertive outreach programs send workers into the community, where they attempt to make consistent contact with these people in order to engage them in treatment and to provide needed services.

Housing is a big problem for the dually diagnosed. Many receive disability payments and are trying to live on meager fixed incomes. Because of the behavior problems associated with addiction, some are evicted from government-supported housing and shelters. Some communities provide supervised group homes for the dually diagnosed where treatment can be monitored and services provided for both kinds of problems.

The challenge to clinicians who treat the dually diagnosed is the diversity of the problems that clients encounter. The severity of the mental illness and of the addiction can range from mild to severe. The majority of people who have addiction and another psychiatric diagnosis are able to participate fully in traditional alcohol and drug programming with only minor modification. But for those with severe mental illness as well as addiction, a spectrum of services is needed to cover all aspects of the person's life.

Outcome measures are clear, and this is the good news. People with severe mental illness and addiction make steady progress in these programs, achieving both recovery from the addiction and more stable remission from the mental illness.

# 9. Gambling, Sex, and Other Addictions

### Addiction or Compulsion?

Several behavioral problems that are closely related to drug and alcohol addiction are viewed as addictions themselves. As we continue to formulate a comprehensive definition of what addiction is, these disorders provide salient examples of why we cannot look to the pharmacological properties of drugs alone as the cause of addiction.

The three most commonly seen conditions that resemble alcohol and drug addiction are pathological gambling, sexual addiction, and eating disorders. Since each of these is characterized by loss of control of the behavior and continued involvement in it despite negative consequences, we view them as addictions.

The cost to society of these three problems is enormous. A 1993 estimate placed the amount of money spent on *legal* gambling at over $300 billion a year. Sexual addiction leads to broken families, AIDS and its medical costs, sexual crimes, and millions spent on pornography. Eating disorders can lead to diabetes, hypertension, and heart disease and even result in sudden death. Millions of dollars are spent each year on weight loss gimmicks. Each of these disorders is also linked to an increased risk of depression and suicide. And the hidden costs—loss of productivity, of well-being, and of self-actualization—can never be measured.

A common misconception is that these behaviors are a manifestation of obsessive-compulsive disorder, since we often describe them as compulsive. Those with obsessive-compulsive disorder have thoughts and urges that seem to come from nowhere and are experienced as odd and anxiety-provoking. These are called obsessions, and usually lead to ritualized behaviors (compulsions) that temporarily reduce the anxiety associated with the thoughts and urges. A person may be obsessed with the danger of contamination and compulsively wash to reduce the risk of being infected. The compulsion results in a relief of anxiety and is intended to avoid the harm predicted by the obsessive thought. In pathological gambling, sex addiction, and eating disorders, the problem lies in the repetitive impulse to engage in a behavior with the goal of obtaining pleasure *despite* possible harmful consequences. It is compulsive in the general sense of the word, but the goal of the behavior is different from what it is in obsessive-compulsive disorder.

These disorders also highlight the behavioral and conditioning aspects of addiction. Behavioral psychologists describe the slot machine as the perfect instrument for illustrating conditioning with variable reinforcement. In this model, the subject engages in a behavior that is known to lead to a reward, but the reward comes at unpredictable intervals. Trainers who want to strongly implant a specific behavioral response in an animal will reward that behavior at intervals rather than every time the animal performs the behavior. As a result, the animal will perform the behavior repeatedly even without a reward. This type of conditioning contributes to gambling addiction. It may be most potent in addiction to video poker games. Gambling counselors have referred to video poker as the crack cocaine of gambling addiction.

Research shows that these disorders also involve activity of the pleasure center of the brain, the ventral tegmentum and medial forebrain bundle. Addiction to alcohol and drugs involves stimulation of this area of the brain by a source outside the body—the drug which is ingested. In behavioral addictions, stimulation of this area of the brain comes from changes in brain chemistry that occur as a result of the addictive behavior. Gambling is thought to stimulate this area through the adrenergic system, sexual addiction through the complex orgasmic response, and eating disorders through the serotoninergic system. In each case, the animal model of repetitive self-stimulation applies.

## Pathological Gambling

The prevalence of pathological gambling is between 1 and 3 percent of the population in the United States. Problem gambling represents roughly another 5 percent. These numbers have risen with the widespread legalization of lotteries and casino gaming. Men outnumber women by a ratio of about two to one. At least half of pathological gamblers are also addicted to alcohol, and studies show that a family history of alcoholism may predispose a person to pathological gambling. Ten percent of the men who are admitted to alcohol and drug treatment meet screening criteria for pathological gambling.

The diagnosis of pathological gambling is based on the presence of several typical patterns of behavior, including gambling to escape stress, spending money that is needed for living expenses, lying about gambling, engaging in illegal acts to obtain money, becoming tolerant to the stimulating effects of gambling, a feeling of restlessness when one is not gambling, and "chasing losses," or betting more in order to cover losses. Problem gamblers are those who may have gambled away needed money or used gambling as a coping strategy but who do not have all of the features asssociated with pathological gambling.

Pathological gambling typically progresses through three stages. First is the winning stage, in which the gambler focuses on how much money is being gained. Self-esteem is linked to winning and to the amount that is won. Next, in the losing stage, the pathological gambler feels insulted and responds as though to a challenge. During this stage, gamblers will begin to chase losses and take inordinate risks with money they can't spare. The desperation stage is third, and involves depletion of resources, complete preoccupation with gambling, and serious psychological consequences. Suicides are common during this phase.

The coexistence of other psychiatric problems is common in pathological gamblers. Major depression is seen in over two-thirds of those identified. Antisocial, narcissistic, and borderline personality disorders are also common.

Pathological gambling is both underrecognized and undertreated. Most gamblers are destitute by the time treatment is sought; many are no longer employed and have no insurance. (Many insurance carriers will not cover treatment for pathological gambling when it is the primary diagnosis even if the gambler still has insurance.) Few professionals are experienced and certified in treating pathological gambling, although their numbers are increasing, especially in states with legalized casino gambling.

Because of the coexistence of depression or alcoholism, pathological gamblers frequently seek treatment in hospital settings. But they often do not recognize or mention that gambling is a problem. Screening for pathological gambling on admission to an alcohol and drug treatment facility or psychiatric hospital is becoming more common, and should probably be routine. The addition of appropriate intervention for the gambling problem can then be provided.

The treatment of pathological gambling is similar to the treatment for other addictions but has some important differences. When the alcoholic or addict goes through "detox" and begins to think clearly, productive changes in attitude often follow. The pathological gambler, however, often does not experience craving and loss of control away from the place where gambling occurs. Discussion of the problem can become merely an intellectual exercise, and no opportunity exists for putting realistic changes into action. Long-term follow-up is therefore essential.

Gamblers Anonymous is a 12-step program based on

Alcoholics Anonymous and can provide ongoing support. GA meetings, however, are not as widely available as AA and NA meetings. Groups facilitated by counselors are helpful but also not widely available. Individual and family therapy is useful, especially in unraveling the secrecy and manipulation associated with the gambling behavior. As problem and pathological gambling become more widespread, treatment centers and government agencies are developing more treatment alternatives.

The presence of major depression is a strong risk factor for the development of pathological gambling and for later relapse. Comprehensive treatment of depression or other coexisting psychiatric problems is essential, as is treatment for any other addictions that might be present, such as alcoholism.

### Sexual Addiction

The *Diagnostic and Statistical Manual* for psychiatric disorders does not list sexual addiction as a specific disorder, but it has been generally recognized as a problem in the psychiatric and addiction literature for many decades.

Compulsive sexual activity meets the criteria for addiction when it involves a loss of control over the behavior and continuation of it despite negative consequences. The particular type of sexual activity may vary and include various behaviors. Some of these behaviors, such as voyeurism and fetishism, are addressed as sexual disorders in the diagnostic manual, and there is some overlap between sexual addiction and other sexual disorders.

The prevalence of sexual addiction in the general population is thought to be between 3 and 6 percent and is more common in men than in women. Sexual addiction often coexists with substance addiction, particularly to cocaine. The prevalence of sexual addiction may be as high as 70 percent in cocaine addicts entering treatment. When unrecognized and untreated, it is a common cause of relapse of the cocaine addiction.

Sexual abuse or inappropriately seductive relationships with adults are common findings in the childhood histories of sex addicts. Sexual abuse damages a child's sense of self and the ability to self-regulate painful emotional states. It also predisposes the child to view sexual activity as a coping strategy. Women with addiction to alcohol or drugs have a higher incidence of sexual addiction than other women, and the prevalence of sexual abuse experienced in the past by women addicts who are in treatment centers has been estimated at about 80 percent.

Treatment of sexual addiction involves a combination of approaches. Twelve-step recovery groups are available and provide useful support. Sex Addicts Anonymous is one such group. Although these groups are generally closed to the public, participation can be gained through referral from a treatment center or a personal interview. Cognitive behavioral psychotherapy is particularly helpful, assisting the individual in identifying core beliefs and basic assumptions that underlie behavioral choices and allowing for conscious changes in behavior. Psychodynamically based psychotherapy is often useful in identifying and addressing the developmental problems that occurred in a person's childhood as a result of abuse.

### Eating Disorders

Eating disorders include anorexia nervosa, bulimia nervosa, and compulsive overeating. Estimates of the prevalence of eating disorders vary among groups of people. They are more common in women than in men and in adolescents and young adults than in older people. The prevalence is higher in cultures that value thinness. Recent surveys found that 1 to 4 percent of white, middle-class female students meet criteria for an eating disorder, and the incidence has been rising for several decades. More cases are being identified in males, often presenting as a preoccupation with body building or exercise.

Eating disorders resemble addiction because they involve a loss of control over the behavior and a continuation of it despite negative consequences. Anorexia nervosa is mentioned because it is an eating disorder, but there are aspects of it that do not resemble an addiction. Classic anorexia nervosa has its onset in childhood or early adolescence and has unique psychological and endocrine characteristics that put it in a class of its own. People with bulimia often go through anorexic phases, particularly during the teen years, and these disorders overlap in some individuals.

Those with eating disorders have a distorted notion of their body image and sense of self. There is frequently a history of trauma and disruption in nurturing relationships during the person's first three years of life and often a history of sexual abuse in childhood as well. People with eating disorders have difficulty with accurately identifying emotions and also physical needs like hunger, as well as with managing painful emotions by themselves. Depression, dissociative disorders, obsessive-compulsive disorder, and borderline personality disorder are commonly seen in people with eating disorders.

Many people with eating disorders have problems with addiction to alcohol and drugs or come from families in which there is addiction. Eating disorders sometimes emerge during early sobriety in recovering alcoholics and addicts.

Bulimia nervosa is characterized by binge eating followed by purging. Purging, or attempting to rid the body of the food eaten during the binge, may take the form of laxative abuse, self-induced vomiting, rigid dieting, or a combination of these behaviors. A loss of control of the binge/purge cycle is typical. The amount of food eaten during a binge can be enormous, sometimes ten thousand calories or more. Cycles may occur in episodes or daily, sometimes several times a day. Often, people with bulimia will steal food or the money to obtain food or laxatives. Massive doses of laxatives are sometimes used, which can lead to malfunction of the colon.

Medical complications are common. Dehydration and electrolyte imbalances occur as a result of the vomiting and diarrhea associated with purging. Despite the massive intake of food, malnutrition is common. Irritation of the throat and destruction of dental enamel is caused by the frequent vomiting. An inability to eat without spontaneous vomiting can also occur. Many women with both anorexia and bulimia stop having menstrual periods. Sudden death due to heart failure or cardiac arrhythmia is a serious risk.

Although compulsive overeating is common, it is not classified as an eating disorder in the *Diagnostic and Statistical Manual*. It is characterized by binge eating but does not involve purging. Compulsive overeaters may be of normal weight, but many are obese. Compulsive overeating shares many psychological features with anorexia and bulimia and often coexists with depression or other psychiatric disorders. (The erroneous belief that compulsive overeating is caused by addiction to sugar is discussed later in this chapter.)

People with eating disorders use food to regulate inner emotional states. Changes in physiology and metabolism associated with the intake of large amounts of food are thought to have a calming effect. The ability to detect actual hunger and satiety is often absent.

The treatment of eating disorders involves a combination of approaches. The behavior must be addressed, but underlying psychological issues must be dealt with as well if lasting change is to occur. Psychodynamically based individual psychotherapy is often helpful. An arrest in early development underlies the distorted notions of body image and problems with self-regulation. Memories associated with this developmental arrest are often preverbal, taking the form of sensations and feelings. The use of expressive therapies including art therapy and psychodrama are useful, as are techniques such as videotaping and working with a mirror in order to develop a sense of one's body shape. Hospitalization may be needed to help a person restore body weight and achieve some control over the disorder. Group support and therapy both in the hospital and after discharge are also helpful.

❋

### Abuse of Anabolic Steroids

Anabolic steroids are hormones that promote the development of muscle tissue. Testosterone is an anabolic steroid that is produced naturally by the gonads and adrenal glands and is responsible for masculine traits. Compounds related to testosterone were first synthesized in the 1930s and since then have been believed by some to promote athletic performance and the development of muscle strength and size. The medical literature, however, has not consistently supported this belief.

Anabolic steroids are used primarily by athletes and body builders. Males use them more commonly than females, by about a ten-to-one ratio. The actual prevalence of steroid abuse is not known, but some surveys have shown that up wards of 50 percent of athletes and 95 percent of body builders have used these drugs at one time or another. Use by teenagers and even preteenagers has been reported.

The abuse of anabolic steroids fits the working definition of addiction because users report a loss of control over the behavior and a continuation of use despite undesired physical consequences. A withdrawal syndrome characterized by depression, loss of sex drive, fatigue, restlessness, and craving has been described. Users often report taking more of the drug and using it over longer periods of time than they intended to, preoccupation with obtaining and using the drug, and significant impairment in their social and occupational functioning as a result of using it.

On the other hand, there are some characteristics of anabolic steroid abuse that differ from alcohol or drug addiction. For example, the initial motivation for using anabolic steroids is the belief that they will enhance physical appearance and athletic performance over time, whereas the motivation to use alcohol and drugs involves immediate change in mood. Anabolic steroid users are typically health conscious, and, before the onset of the abuse, often avoid alcohol or drugs.

Over the last several decades public awareness of the dangers of anabolic steroid abuse has increased. Most amateur, collegiate, and professional athletic associations have banned the use of these drugs and test for their presence in athletes. Government oversight of the production and distribution of anabolic steroids has decreased the quantities that are diverted to illicit use, but the availability of foreign and illegally produced steroids has increased.

Anabolic steroids are typically taken in cycles of several weeks, during which the doses increase in a preset pattern that users call a pyramid. At the end of the cycle, the total dose may be many times the usual medical dose. Some athletes do only one or two cycles and stop. Those who complete at least five cycles are at higher risk for addiction. Adverse effects of anabolic steroid use are both psychological and physical. The drug can cause irritability, aggressiveness, depression, and paranoia. (As many as two-thirds of heavy users have reported acting aggressively while under its influence.) Physical toxicity includes liver damage and jaundice, high blood pressure, strokes, premature baldness, reduced testicular size, and low sperm counts.

Steroid receptors are found in several areas of the brain that are involved in the control and regulation of emotion. It is thought that overstimulation of these areas by massive doses of anabolic steroids and their metabolites may not only contribute to the psychological effects but may also increase levels of endogenous opiates. This may be the mechanism by which loss of control, withdrawal symptoms, and cravings occur.

Anabolic steroid users frequently abuse other drugs for a

variety of purposes. Other hormones may be taken to counteract the undesired physical effects, and mood-altering drugs may be used to counteract the psychological effects. Because the user is thereby introduced to mood-altering drugs and to the drug culture, anabolic steroids are considered to be gateway drugs.

There is also some overlap between anabolic steroid abuse and eating disorders. Although once considered rare in males, bulimia nervosa has been identified in body builders and athletes, some of whom also abuse anabolic steroids.

### What Else Constitutes Addiction?

A number of other behaviors and kinds of substance use are commonly referred to as addictions. These include excessive time spent on computer games, the Internet, TV sports, and golf, compulsive shopping, and "workaholism." Some people believe that sugar and chocolate have specific addictive qualities and are the cause of compulsive overeating.

If we go back to the basic definition of addiction—that it involves loss of control over the use of a substance (or the practice of a behavior) and the inability to stop despite negative consequences—then we can consider at least some of these perhaps to have the characteristics of addiction.

Recent studies of compulsive computer users identify characteristics including preoccupation with use of the machine, restlessness when one is not using it, a continuation of use despite physical consequences such as carpal tunnel syndrome or eye strain, and neglect of job and family responsibilities. Some of those studied had addiction to drugs and alcohol and were abstinent at the time when the computer use became a problem. Some computer use, such as chat room participation and Internet pornography, overlaps with sexual addiction. A number of users were preoccupied with computer games, which may have the same reinforcing qualities found in slot machines or video poker, although without the anticipation of monetary gain.

Compulsive shopping has also been characterized as an addiction since it involves financial consequences and loss of control. Compulsive shoppers are usually women, and some are also addicted to drugs and alcohol. They consciously use shopping as a mood-altering activity, believing that buying something will make them feel better and being disappointed when it doesn't work.

There is some overlap between compulsive shopping and eating disorders. From a dynamic standpoint, the aim of the behavior is similar—satisfaction of a vague emotional neediness. This is followed by the subconscious realization that purchasing items at a store is only a symbolic substitute and does not satisfy the emotional need. It is believed that, for those with eating disorders, this cycle represents an unconscious attempt to re-create the frustrating relationship with early caregivers.

Excessive shopping is sometimes seen during the manic or hypomanic phases of bipolar disorder. In this situation the behavior is a reflection of impaired judgment and grandiosity and is not the same as compulsive shopping. Kleptomania, or compulsive shop*lifting*, is classified as a disorder of impulse control. In a general sense it could be considered an addiction, but it's viewed by clinicians as a reflection of a deeper disturbance in personality functioning that goes beyond the dynamics of addiction.

Hoarding is a symptom of obsessive-compulsive disorder that may involve excessive shopping. The term refers to a person's inability to throw away items of little value, which may include old newspapers and magazines, rubber bands, jars, junk mail, and worn-out clothing. Sometimes items of little apparent value are purchased in large quantities and saved, often in their original bags. People who have experienced poverty and deprivation often appear to be pathological hoarders, but the difference lies in the approach to cleaning

up the mess that ensues. For those who suffer from pathological hoarding, throwing out or giving things away causes
intense anxiety, whereas people from poor backgrounds are
able to make rational decisions about what goes or stays.

We often refer to preoccupation with such activities as
watching TV sports, following soap operas, playing golf,
talking on the phone, reading romance or mystery novels,
collecting dolls, and going to garage sales as addictions. People may engage in these practices to excess in order to cope
with emotional stress and to gain satisfaction. What seems
like an addiction to a family member—for example, to a "golf
widow"—may actually constitute behavior that reflects some
problem the person is having, with the marital relationship
or otherwise. Defining and then treating these behaviors as
"addictions" may miss the point entirely.

On the other hand, engaging excessively in a particular
behavior is often seen in people who have addiction and are
currently abstinent. What has happened is that the addict has
begun to use a specific behavior to cope with uncomfortable
feelings, rather than continuing to learn to identify and resolve these feelings in an effective manner. This is often an
early symptom of relapse. I frequently see "workaholism"
in addicts who later relapse. They throw themselves into
work as a way of coping with the stress of recovery and to
recoup the financial losses associated with the addiction.
Continued growth stops and the addict begins to lose sight
of the principles of recovery. The person in recovery turns
into a "dry drunk," and many eventually "wet it down" by
relapsing because they are not experiencing the contentment
and satisfaction that comes with true recovery. Such behavior
problems occurring in recovering people should not be seen
as a new addiction but as a reason for returning to work on
the original one.

The chocolate question is an interesting one. Chocolate
contains a compound that may have psychoactive qualities.
Informal studies have suggested that when we eat chocolate,

we feel as though we are in love—hence the custom of giving chocolate for Valentine's Day. Addicts in recovery love chocolate. (There is a scene in the movie *Clean and Sober* that always gets a laugh when it's shown at a treatment center. One of the characters is on pass from a treatment center and spends his time sitting on the side of his bed eating mounds of Hershey's Kisses.) Some compulsive overeaters report specific cravings for chocolate. However there is little evidence that a chocolate "addiction" occurs if we apply the criterion that addiction must cause significant impairment in functioning or emotional distress.

The belief that sugar is addicting to compulsive overeaters has a large following, especially among compulsive overeaters in recovery, but there is little scientific evidence to support such a notion. I believe that this phenomenon is due to the difficulty compulsive overeaters have in identifying what abstinence means for them and what the addiction really is. Targeting sugar as the culprit provides a concrete solution.

Abstaining from eating—as opposed to abstaining from drinking alcohol or using drugs—is obviously not the solution. Neither is dieting, since many compulsive overeaters are also compulsive dieters. The obesity that results from compulsive overeating is a secondary effect and not the primary problem, but the social discomfort and damage to self-esteem that obesity causes makes losing weight a priority. Abstinence from compulsive overeating really involves using food only for nutritional sustenance and not as a way of altering mood, but this does not always result in the desired weight loss.

Strict abstinence from any food that contains refined sugar, which includes most breads, pastas, condiments, and processed foods, is sometimes recommended at Overeaters Anonymous meetings. Members who swear off sugar sometimes report "withdrawal" symptoms, such as headaches, lethargy, and irritability, early on. And following this type of regimen does result in weight loss. *Sugar Busters* is a popular diet book based on the concept that intake of refined sugar leads to impaired metabolism and subsequent obesity.

What we do know is that intake of refined sugar causes sharp increases in circulating levels of insulin. That is because refined sugar is quickly absorbed and blood sugar levels rise quickly. One of the functions of insulin is to regulate blood sugar levels by causing glucose to be converted to fat and then stored. But the pancreas often "overshoots" because of the sharp rise in blood sugar, and this leads to a rebound effect resulting in a sharp drop in blood sugar that motivates the person to eat again. If the person becomes obese, fat cells enlarge and become more resistant to the effects of insulin. As a result, the pancreas produces even more insulin, which promotes more fat storage and a greater rebound when refined sugar is eaten. The effect is more pronounced in people who are genetically predisposed to adult-onset diabetes mellitus.

Complex carbohydrates break down more slowly than refined sugar and therefore do not cause sharp increases in circulating insulin levels. The ups and downs of blood sugar do not occur, so that the motivation to overeat decreases. Compulsive overeaters who abstain from refined carbohydrates may feel an increased sense of control over their food intake, but the psychological dynamics of the eating disorder still need to be addressed.

Since this complex metabolic effect occurs only as a result of the overeating and subsequent obesity, I can't agree with its being characterized as addiction to sugar. The eating disorder arises from the difficulty a compulsive overeater has in self-regulation and self-soothing and from the mood-altering effects of food intake on the emotional centers of the brain. Any food, not just refined sugar, can have this effect.

# 10. The Search for a Cure

In the past several decades our understanding of addiction and its many aspects has increased at a tremendous rate. We now know that addiction is a complex disorder involving several chemical systems in the brain and that the brains of addicts function in an abnormal manner. We have seen that genes play an important role in a person's vulnerability to addiction. We have also seen that social factors, conditioning, emotional elements, and the characteristics of the drugs themselves contribute to the disease of addiction.

Great strides have been made in the development of effective treatments for addiction. Until the mid-1960s, hospital treatment for alcoholism and drug dependence was almost nonexistent and often consisted simply of medical detoxification and advice that the person stop drinking or using drugs. We now have more effective therapies and medications that help the addict recover.

But there is much work left to be done. Current research targets several different areas, including the following: (1) epidemiology—tracking the prevalence and types of addictions and who is affected, (2) genetics—identifying addiction genes to discover who is at risk, (3) pharmacology—understanding more fully how addictive drugs work and developing new medications to counteract the effects of addiction, and (4) treatment—devising and testing treatment strategies and measuring outcomes.

## Epidemiology

The National Institutes of Health and its divisions on alcohol and drug abuse maintain numerous data collection vehicles concerning all aspects of addiction. (Most of these surveys can be readily obtained on the Web sites listed in appendix B.) A few examples of data collected by the National Institute on Alcohol Abuse and Alcoholism (NIAAA) are the National Hospital Discharge Survey (which tracks alcohol-related illness), information on traffic fatalities and blood alcohol levels provided by the National Highway Traffic Safety Administration and related agencies, alcohol consumption data from state alcohol agencies and the alcoholic beverage industry, and the National Longitudinal Alcohol Epidemiological Survey. A comprehensive listing of current survey reports and the reports themselves can be obtained directly from NIAAA.

The National Institute on Drug Abuse (NIDA) maintains several sources of surveillance data, including the Drug Abuse Warning Network (DAWN) composed of selected emergency rooms, medical examiners, crisis centers, and other agencies. DAWN tracks illnesses and deaths believed to be the result of addiction and is often able to provide early indications of new trends in drug abuse such as the recent resurgence of heroin addiction. Prescription audits and recapture studies by the Drug Enforcement Administration also provide useful data. (Recapture studies were first done to gather information on wildlife. When an animal is captured, it is measured and tagged, and when recaptured it is measured again.) Identified contacts within the drug community are tracked, and their activities provide useful information about trends in substance abuse. The National Institute of Justice conducts an ongoing survey of arrestees at selected urban sites across the country called the Arrestee Drug Abuse Monitoring Program (ADAM). Data is collected quarterly and includes both an interview and a urine drug screen. The United Nations also tracks several sources of data through its various agencies, including WHO and UNESCO.

The Substance Abuse and Mental Health Services Administration (SAMHSA) of the U.S. Department of Health and Human Services conducts the annual National Household

Survey on Drug Abuse. Use of alcohol and drugs over the past month, past year, and person's lifetime is tracked and analyzed. State and local agencies use this survey in order to design and implement more detailed surveillance. The Household Survey provides data relevant to community prevention groups, to legislatures, to agencies planning health care delivery systems, and to law enforcement.

Survey data in 1998 revealed that 13.6 million Americans were current users of illicit drugs (use within thirty days) and that 4.1 million met diagnostic criteria for drug addiction. Of those addicted, 1.1 million were between the ages of twelve and seventeen. One hundred thirteen million Americans had drunk alcohol within the past thirty days, and 10.5 million were between the ages of twelve and twenty. Twelve million were described as heavy drinkers. Survey data also confirmed the observation of addiction professionals that the use of heroin and hallucinogens is on the rise. First time use of heroin in youths has risen to levels not seen since the early 1970s. First time hallucinogen use by those between the ages of twelve and seventeen rose during the 1990s, with 1.1 million new users in 1997.

In 1994 and 1997 the Household Survey contained questions about drug and alcohol use in the workplace. It was noted that 70 percent of current drug users were employed, with 7.7 percent of full-time employees reporting current illicit drug use and about the same number reporting heavy drinking. Data was also gathered on occupation, sex, ethnic group, workplace drug testing, and other variables.

Critical to those who plan and provide funding for prevention and treatment are studies that look at the costs of addiction to society. These cost-of-illness studies are complex and cover three main areas of inquiry: what the connection is between addiction and various adverse outcomes such as medical and social problems, to what degree addiction is directly responsible for these outcomes, and how to determine what the cost is to society. The studies draw upon the diverse surveillance data provided by the kinds of surveys mentioned above, using information from the health care industry and from death reports, workplace data, household surveys, correctional facilities, law enforcement, welfare agencies, transportation safety agencies, and fire departments. "Opportunity cost" determines the value of resources that are diverted from one use to another because of addiction problems. Costs of direct health care are measured and an estimate made of lost productivity resulting from addiction. Additional costs associated with crime, accidents, and other alcohol- and drug-related events are also measured.

A comprehensive cost-of-illness study released by the National Institutes of Health in 1998 placed the annual cost of alcohol and drug abuse at $246 billion, or $965 per capita. Of these costs, roughly 60 percent had to do with alcohol and 40 percent with drugs. Compared to figures in the last cost-of-illness study done in the 1980s, costs had risen substantially, even when factors such as changes in methodology were considered, largely because of a higher level of drug abuse and addiction following the late 1970s. The crack cocaine epidemic of the 1980s and the sharp rise in drug-related crime were responsible for a substantial percentage of the increase in costs.

### Genetics

Genetics research includes not only examination of the patterns of inheritance in families but also direct examination of the genes themselves. Advances in molecular biology have allowed researchers to literally break open a chromosome and examine the coding that determines our genetic traits. The ability to alter the gene structure of experimental animals has led to testing of the function and importance of specific genes, sometimes with unexpected results.

A primary aim is to determine who is vulnerable to addiction and why. An ongoing study by Dr. Mark Schuckit at the University of California at San Diego is tracking several

traits in three generations of men initially selected for study
in the mid-1970s. Findings so far confirm the "low response"
factor seen in the sons of alcoholics. Those sons were later re-
contacted and found to be three times more likely to develop
alcoholism than those in the general population. Beginning
in 1999 a third generation was added to the study. As these
children grow up, several variables will be measured to see
if it is possible to predict the risk of alcoholism and target
specific traits for prevention and early intervention. This
valuable cohort group of almost fifteen hundred subjects also
provides a potential source of data for more detailed genetic
analysis.

Family studies on the genetics of drug dependence are also
under way. Dr. Kathleen Merikangas and her colleagues at
Yale University recently published an analysis of the families
of almost three hundred individuals with drug dependence.
Their findings confirmed that the presence of addiction to a
particular substance elevates risk for addiction to that substance in family members. Studies such as these provide a
focus for more detailed inquiry into the genetics of specific
drug addictions.

The amount of research on drug addiction has lagged
behind research on alcoholism because of differences in
funding patterns and political interest. Sharp increases in
the prevalence and cost of drug dependence documented
by epidemiological surveys have led, though, to increased
support for research on the various aspects of illicit drug
addiction.

The DNA molecule is composed of interlocking strands
of molecules set up like a twisting ladder. The rungs of the
ladder are composed of pairs of four different molecules
in different combinations. Each individual has a unique se-
quence of these four molecules, since no two individuals share
identical genetic characteristics unless they are identical twins.
However, there are stretches of DNA which code specific
characteristics (hair or eye color, for example) that will be

the same for different groups of individuals. DNA molecules
are found in the chromosomes, which are x-shaped structures
found in the nucleus of the cell. Each chromosome contains
details concerning the structure and function of a particular
part of the body. The first step in understanding genetics was
to discover what genes—or groups of DNA molecules—are
contained in which chromosome. We are now able to untwist
the DNA molecules that form the genes and figure out what
combinations of the ladder's rungs correspond to a particular
genetic trait.

There are several basic approaches to the study of the
genetics of a particular condition. The first of these is linkage
analysis. In this type of study the genes of affected individuals
are compared to the genes of family members with and without related disorders to see if patterns cluster in certain areas
of the chromosome. Very simply put, the DNA is unwound
and compared so as to determine whether there are specific
repeating patterns that can be identified in people with the
disease in question. In allele-sharing studies the genes of
people from the same family with the same condition are
compared. Again, patterns that recur are identified as possible
sites that control the expression of the disease in question.

Association studies compare the genes of those who have
the disorder to the genes of those who don't. A particular
pattern of genes that consistently shows up in people with
the disorder, but not in those without it, is considered to be
associated with the disorder. Proceeding further in the lab
to identify what characteristic that gene controls helps us
to understand what causes the disorder. Often in this type
of study something as subtle as a slight difference in the
structure of a single enzyme is found.

In the fourth type of study strains of experimental animals with specifically bred traits are compared. One type
of experimental animal is called a "knock-out" animal. Its
genes are altered in the lab so that a specific gene at a specific
location is removed. This is generally the gene that controls a

characteristic that has already been identified and is suspected of being involved in the disorder being studied. As a result of this genetic manipulation the animal does not express the traits controlled by that gene. When these animals are exposed to a particular drug or some other experimental condition, their response can be compared to the response of animals who have an intact set of genes. This gives the researcher more detailed information on what that gene does by observing what happens when it is absent.

The National Institute on Alcohol Abuse and Alcoholism has recently published initial findings from an extensive multicenter project called the Collaborative Study on the Genetics of Alcoholism (COGA), centered at the State University of New York Downstate College of Medicine in Brooklyn. A sister study, also extensively examining the genetics of alcoholism, is under way at NIAAA headquarters in Rockville, Maryland.

In a linkage study of decreased brain wave activity in response to electrical stimulation (P3 event related potentials), COGA researchers found linkages on chromosomes 2 and 6 and possible linkages on chromosomes 5 and 13. P3 event related potentials are an interesting phenomenon. An event related potential is a positive brain wave that occurs following some type of sensory stimulation. A spike occurs three hundred milliseconds after a novel stimulus, and this is called a "P3" potential. For reasons that are not entirely clear, sons of male alcoholics demonstrate a lower amplitude of this type of brain wave. Since low P3 amplitude has been consistently associated with the risk for alcoholism, this study helps pinpoint sites for more detailed analysis.

An allele-sharing study of almost one thousand people from families affected by alcoholism found that the risk for alcoholism might involve traits controlled by genes on chromosomes 1, 2, and 7. Further evidence for the protective effect from the development of alcoholism on chromosome 4 was also presented. This protective effect involves the enzyme alcohol dehydrogenase and has been the focus of research in other settings. Alcohol dehydrogenase is an enzyme involved in the metabolism of alcohol. People with a certain form of this enzyme do not metabolize alcohol as efficiently as others, and will experience an unpleasant flushing reaction after ingesting alcohol.

COGA study data is presently being made available to researchers at other facilities, and its work continues as well. A prospective study of the children in the original group is planned to see which children develop problems with alcohol. Further study of their genetic characteristics will provide valuable information.

The NIAAA study confirmed the finding of the protective effect on chromosome 4 related to the alcohol dehydrogenase gene. Previous family studies had suggested that this effect was limited to Asians who experience an unpleasant flushing sensation when drinking alcohol. But these and other studies suggest that a more subtle effect may be present in other racial groups. The exact mechanism of the protective effect is still under study.

Another finding of the NIAAA study identified a linkage with a specific portion of chromosome 11 in people genetically at risk for alcoholism. Chromosome 11 has been identified as containing genes that control the synthesis of neurotransmitters important in addiction, such as serotonin and dopamine. This is an example of how a linkage study, combined with previous research findings, points the way towards further study.

Two recent studies with knock-out animals have increased our understanding of the actions of cocaine. Researchers at NIDA bred knock-out mice which lacked a specific receptor for the neurotransmitter serotonin—5HT(1b). These mice, when compared to their unaffected cousins, were more sensitive to the effects of cocaine and more strongly attracted to the drug. 5HT(1b) knock-out mice also react more strongly to alcohol and are more impulsive. Their response to different experimental situations with different drugs should prove helpful in our understanding of the molecular mechanisms behind addiction.

The second study, also coming out of NIDA, found an unexpected connection between a sensitization response to cocaine and the lack of a gene that controls the biological clock. This study used knock-out strains of fruit flies, which have some genetic similarity to humans. The gene knocked out in the fruit flies was the one regulating the biological clock, a timing device that controls various bodily processes occurring cyclically over time. Sensitization to a drug like cocaine is manifested by an increased response to its effects after repeated exposures. This was blunted in the fruit flies that lacked the clock gene. The implication of this finding is not yet clear, but it opens up a new area of potential inquiry that should prove helpful in furthering our understanding of how the brain responds to cocaine and other drugs.

Knock-out mice were used in a recent study of nicotine addiction. In this study, mice were bred so as to lack a component of the nicotinic acetylcholine receptor in the brain, a receptor for the neurotransmitter acetylcholine which also binds nicotine. These knock-out mice did not self-administer nicotine, unlike their unaffected cohorts. Since self-administration is a component of drug addiction, it was concluded that this receptor subunit must be involved in the addictive properties of nicotine. Another study found that people who inherit the less-active variant of a common liver enzyme, CYP2A6, which metabolizes nicotine and other drugs, were less likely to develop addiction to nicotine. This might help explain why some people become addicted to nicotine more easily than others.

## Pharmacology

Studies on the pharmacology of addiction focus on the properties of addictive drugs as they interact with the brain and on potential drug treatments for addiction. Some of this research overlaps with genetic research, as, for example, in studies using knock-out mice. The use of noninvasive brain imaging techniques such as positron emission tomography (PET) and functional magnetic resonance imaging (fMRI) allows researchers to watch how the brain responds to doses of a drug.

Researchers at Harvard used fMRI to study how the brain responds as a person experiences a dose of cocaine. This novel technique opens up a new area of potential research. We are now able to watch what happens to the brain during the various phases of drug use. Different parts of the brain were activated during these phases. For example, the cortex and limbic system were activated during the initial "rush," but at times, when subjects reported feelings of craving, the nucleus accumbens was activated. The nucleus accumbens is part of the pleasure center of the brain that has been implicated in the reinforcing properties of addictive drugs.

Another study of cocaine involved the use of knock-out mice which lacked genes responsible for the movement of serotonin and dopamine in and out of cells. It was previously thought that these neurotransmitters were responsible for the addictive activation of the pleasure center of the brain. But the mice continued to show a preference for cocaine. What this study indicates is that there is a broader and more complex reaction to cocaine that underlies its addictive qualities.

PET scanning was recently used to compare the reinforcing effects of stimulants in people with low and high levels of dopamine $D_2$ receptors, which are involved in the experience of euphoria when a person is using amphetamines. People with low $D_2$ levels were more likely to experience euphoria with a dose of an amphetamine. People with high $D_2$ levels tended to dislike the stimulant effect. This study increases our understanding of why some people are more likely than others to become addicted to amphetamines.

Electrical self-stimulation of the brain's pleasure center and rates of self-administration by laboratory animals are commonly used to study the addictive potential of various drugs. In this paradigm, electrodes that stimulate the brain's pleasure center when activated are placed in the animal's brain. Using the electrical self-stimulation paradigm, Athina Markou and colleagues at the Scripps Institute in La Jolla, California, measured the rate of electrical self-stimulation in rats before and after cessation of nicotine use. The rats were stabilized on nicotine doses equivalent to those of a typical smoker. After the nicotine was stopped, the rats needed a substantial increase in the intensity of the electrical stimulation. This finding suggests that nicotine withdrawal is associated with a decrease in the brain's ability to feel pleasure. Similar results occur during withdrawal from other addictive drugs. The ability to pinpoint the site in the brain responsible for the unpleasant symptoms of withdrawal could lead to more effective drug therapy.

Currently, few medications are effective in treating addiction, and that is a major focus of research. As we learn more about the molecular mechanisms involved in addiction, the development of new drugs becomes possible. At present, most drugs being studied for use in addiction are those that have already been developed for another purpose.

These drugs are used in experimental trials and their effects analyzed. Drug trials are of two main types—open-label and blinded. In open-label studies both the researcher and the subject know what drug is being administered and why. This type of study helps researchers decide whether there is a possibility that the drug might be useful. But further testing is needed, since it is not possible in an open-label trial to know whether there was a true drug effect or whether it was a placebo effect, which is common with psychoactive drugs. A placebo effect is a positive response based on a psychological reaction rather than on the workings of the drug. To rule out a placebo response and to make sure that the findings in an open trial are not just coincidence, a more rigorous blinded study is done, which involves concealing the identity of the drug from the subject or the researcher or both. The purpose of the drug is known, but some of the subjects are intentionally given another drug or a placebo as a basis of comparison. Only after the study is completed does the researcher know who received the drug in question and who did not.

Opiate receptor blockers have shown promise in the treatment of alcoholism and addiction to opiates. These medications, which have been used for many years in emergency rooms to treat overdoses, literally push the drug off the receptor and reverse its effects. Naltrexone has been shown to reduce the frequency of relapse in opiate addicts and has been commercially available for several years. What is intriguing, however, is that studies have shown a similar benefit in alcoholics, and the use of naltrexone in the treatment of alcoholism is now well accepted in clinical practice. A related drug called nalmefene also shows promise in reducing relapse rates in alcoholics. Nalmefene differs from naltrexone in that it targets more than one opioid receptor.

Drugs that block the cravings associated with cocaine use are being actively sought; a number that are currently available have shown promise in open trials in reducing such cravings. Among these are the antidepressants imipramine and fluoxetine and the mood stabilizers carbamezepine and valproate. Studies in which a blinded methodology was used have not, however, consistently supported their effectiveness. A drug that works consistently to reduce cravings will provide a breakthrough in the treatment of addiction.

### Treatment Approaches and Outcomes

Another major focus of addiction research is on the development and measurement of effective psychosocial treatment and follow-up studies of the long-term outcomes of different approaches. The Drug Abuse Treatment Outcome Studies project was initiated by NIDA in the early 1990s. This project involves four centers—the National Development and Research Institutes in North Carolina, Texas Christian University in Ft. Worth, Texas, the University of California at Los Angeles, and the NIDA Services Research Branch in Maryland. Data on over ten thousand addicts who received treatment in four types of settings has been collected with long-term follow-up planned over the next four years on roughly a third of the original sample. These settings include outpatient methadone clinics, long-term residential treatment, drug-free outpatient programs, and short-term inpatient treatment. Data from the study is available from the Substance Abuse and Mental Health Data Archive (SAMHDA) at the University of Michigan.

The Substance Abuse and Mental Health Services Administration (SAMHSA) of the U.S. Department of Health and Human Services makes available a number of services for treatment providers and also coordinates nationwide treatment-outcome studies. The Center for Substance Abuse Treatment (CSAT) is a division of SAMHSA that collects and disseminates state-of-the-art information concerning all aspects of addiction treatment. The National Treatment Improvement Evaluation Study (NTIES) is a recent treatment-outcome survey that looked at patient characteristics and types of treatment settings to determine factors that favored a positive outcome. Completion of the entire treatment program, higher intensity of treatment, and longer treatment were associated with better outcomes. The specific characteristics of the treatment unit did not explain much of the variation, nor did more severe addiction at the time of admission.

SAMHSA also supports an ongoing study called TOPPS, which stands for Treatment Outcomes and Performance Pilot Studies. This nationwide study, involving participants in fourteen states, is based in publicly supported treatment programs administered at the state level. Each state has identified target areas for study within the populations that they serve. The findings of the TOPPS project will be a compilation of a number of studies covering different outcome and treatment issues. Some areas of interest include the effect of managed care on treatment outcomes and the assessment of approaches used with various ethnic and cultural groups.

Contingency management is a recently studied therapeutic technique used in the treatment of cocaine addiction. In this approach behavioral reinforcement is based on the addict's performance in treatment. The intention is to help counteract the classical conditioning that results in cravings for cocaine when the addict is exposed to an environment where drugs are being used. Vouchers that can be redeemed for retail merchandise are given to addicts in outpatient treatment who have negative urine drug screens. In one randomized trial, addicts assigned to the voucher program showed better treatment retention rates and longer periods of abstinence than those in standard treatment.

Cognitive behavioral therapy involves a supportive and educative approach that teaches the addict to identify core beliefs underlying problem behaviors and to make better choices about drug use. Cognitive behavioral theory is also the basis of relapse prevention protocols which have been added to most treatment programs, and has been applied to couples and family therapy strategies. The addition of cognitive behavioral treatment to traditional treatment approaches has been shown to enhance treatment outcome.

Harm reduction is another treatment approach that has been found to work well with addicts who also have a diagnosis of severe mental illness. This is a treatment paradigm that diverges from the previous belief that total abstinence is the definition of positive outcome. Harm reduction measures such elements as the length of time between using and abstaining and the degree of negative consequences associated with the addiction. The eventual goal of a harm reduction protocol is still abstinence, but it allows for gradual progress as the addict with mental illness becomes more engaged over time in the treatment process.

In summary, research on addiction is varied and plentiful, which, considering the immense complexity of the condition, is not surprising. Much more material is available than what I have discussed here. Interested readers can contact NIAAA, NIDA, SAMHSA, and the NIH directly by mail or phone or by accessing the Web sites provided in appendix B. The *American Journal on Addictions* (only one of several journals featuring articles on addiction) is published quarterly by the American Psychiatric Association Press and includes new research on many different topics.

As we explore the intricacies of the addicted brain, perhaps we will unlock some of the secrets of how that organ functions and how it integrates thoughts, memories, feelings, hopes, aspirations, and spirituality to form the essence of what we call human nature.

A quotation from *Alcoholics Anonymous* (the Big Book) seems appropriate here: "Physicians who are familiar with alcoholism agree there is no such thing as making a normal drinker out of an alcoholic. Science may one day accomplish this, but it hasn't done so yet." Actually, anyone who has attained true sobriety and along with it a sense of contentment and serenity doesn't really care if science ever accomplishes that. Such a person no longer feels the need to be a normal drinker.

# Appendix A: Regulation of Addictive Substances

The United States has made various social and legislative attempts to deal with addiction, especially in the twentieth century. But history reflects our society's ambivalence about whether to outlaw addictive substances or to allow and regulate the consumption of them. Efforts to ban the use and sale of alcohol during Prohibition led to the growth of an underground black market and organized crime. When it was believed that heroin addiction was the cause of increasing inner-city crime in the 1940s and 1950s, heroin addicts were listed on federal registers and sent to federal treatment centers. The advent of methadone maintenance treatment, controversial as it was, allowed heroin addicts to reenter society but made little impact on the course of the addiction itself in the individual addict.

In the 1960s the use of hallucinogens for their "mind expanding" powers was promoted by some, and legislation was passed to decriminalize the possession and use of marijuana. The subsequent epidemic of crack cocaine use, however, increased public concern about the destructive aspects of drug addiction, and vast amounts of tax dollars have been spent on the "war on drugs." When AIDS became epidemic among intravenous drug users, proponents of clean needle programs came forward, but so did people who strongly opposed those programs. We have seen increasing social concern about drunk driving, but attempts to lower the legal alcohol blood limit nationally have engendered controversy. And while some debate the regulation of nicotine products, including cigarettes, others promote the easing of restrictions on casino gambling.

Before the early 1900s, unregulated sale of patent medicines led to widespread opiate addiction. In the 1800s most pharmacies sold preparations such as Dover's Powder and McMunn's Elixir of Opium, which contained morphine. Derivatives of the coca plant including extracts and pure cocaine were widely used for their stimulant properties and were not considered harmful. Coca-Cola is an example of a popular tonic that contained active cocaine when it was first produced. Some acknowledgment of the addicting nature of these patent medicines was made in the medical and religious literature, but social disapproval of their use was minimal.

In the early 1900s the federal government instituted control over the sale and use of opiates. The Pure Food and Drug Act of 1906 required that all patent medicines have an accurate list of ingredients, conform to standards of purity, and truthfully describe their intended effects. Public awareness of the extent of the availability of opiates increased, and educational efforts were made to reduce the prevalence of addiction to these tonics.

The Shanghai Opium Commission was convened under the leadership of Theodore Roosevelt and led to the adoption of the Smoking Opium Exclusion Act of 1909. The Hague Treaty of 1911 called for national and international efforts to curb the use and distribution of opium and coca products. These actions stemmed from the conflict in the Far East over the opium trade and the international recognition of a need to control and monitor the production and distribution of narcotics, including the "tonics" that contained opiates.

The Harrison Narcotics Act of 1914 was a landmark in government regulation of addictive substances. It was followed by a series of revisions and further regulations that instituted and strengthened federal government control of the possession, distribution, and use of opiates and cocaine. The prohibition of alcohol began in 1919 following ratification of the Eighteenth Amendment by all but two states. Marijuana came under federal control following the Marihuana [sic] Tax Act of 1937.

At the present time, no fewer than twenty-two federal agencies play a role in the implementation of federal drug policy and participate in the Demand Reduction Working

Group, which is charged with implementing aspects of the National [drug] Strategy that deals with the problem of addiction itself. The government also directs efforts at reducing the drug supply and at coordinating state and federal activities through the Office of National Drug Control Policy, which was created in the late 1980s.

The Drug Enforcement Administration (DEA) was established in 1973. It grew out of the Narcotics Division of the Treasury Department's Internal Revenue Bureau, which was created in 1919 to enforce alcohol prohibition, and the Federal Bureau of Narcotics, which was established in 1930. This regulatory department merged with the law enforcement agency known as the Office of Drug Abuse Law Enforcement.

One function of the DEA is the scheduling, or regulation, of addictive substances and the licensing and oversight of the prescribing and dispensing of regulated substances. These substances include most of those known to cause problems with addiction, with the exception of alcohol. A drug is assigned to one of five groups called schedules. The lower the number, the more addictive or problematic the substance. For example, substances found under Schedule I, such as marijuana and heroin, are highly addictive and problematic and have no legal medical use. Substances found under Schedule V, such as paregoric and some cough preparations, have little potential for addiction if used properly.

A major loophole in the law involves substances that can cause addiction but are not scheduled. A drug cannot be scheduled if it is not known to exist, because drugs that are scheduled are specifically identified by their chemical structure. Clever chemists have taken advantage of this loophole by creating "designer drugs"—chemicals closely related to scheduled drugs but technically not illegal. Tragic consequences have resulted from reckless experimentation with these designer drugs. A small change in chemical structure can produce a toxin that mimics an illegal drug. An epidemic of severe Parkinson's disease in young adults was attributed to the production and distribution of such a chemical. Parkinson's disease is a degenerative brain disorder that results in tremors, stiffness, immobility, and loss of mental capacity. A particular designer drug caused permanent brain damage in its users, leaving them crippled and institutionalized.

As we learn more about what makes substances addictive and how to study them in the laboratory, more drugs come to be considered for scheduling. One of these is the compound ephedrine, which is currently available over the counter; it has a chemical structure resembling that of the amphetamines and produces similar effects. Cases of ephedrine abuse and dependence are not uncommon. Ephedrine is also used illegally by chemists to prepare illicit drugs. Another is the muscle relaxer Soma, which was not initially thought of as a drug with potential for abuse, but so many clinicians have seen patients who take advantage of its sedative properties that it has now been recognized as problematic.

Some synthetic drugs were initially marketed because the manufacturers believed that the new chemical structure would be less addicting than the natural compound from which they came. An example of this is pentazocine (Talwin), a potent painkiller that is used following surgery or with painful conditions such as cancer. It was initially thought to be less addictive than natural morphine, which it was meant to replace; however, it quickly joined the ranks of drugs being abused. In the late seventies and early eighties it was popular among drug abusers in the form of "T's and blues," a combination of Talwin and an antihistamine which were melted down and injected.

Some people are of the opinion that just about anything can be abused if it is used to excess, even aspirin or Tylenol. But some drugs that we use for emotional conditions such as depression and psychosis don't seem to have any abuse potential at all. One clever way of monitoring this is to study what the street value is of a drug once it is in general use. Street value is the amount of money an addict will pay for a dose of the drug on the street. So far, all of the classes of drugs that are known to have street value interact in some fashion with the pleasure center of the brain. Drugs that don't do this seem not to develop a street value or to have much potential for misuse or addiction. One study showed that there were some drugs street addicts would pay for and some they would pay *not* to take! The ones they didn't like were drugs that are legitimately used for some psychiatric disorders. People don't become addicted to most of the drugs that are prescribed for emotional and psychiatric conditions.

As a society, we continue to be ambivalent about how to deal with addiction. Cultural attitudes are important, as are legislation and regulation, but in the end the solution lies with individual choice. Attention to mental problems such as depression, anxiety, and psychological trauma, support from families and friends, and the expectation that each individual will assume personal responsibility for making choices are social factors that favor a reduction in the prevalence of addiction. As we develop more effective treatments and increase our awareness of addiction and its many manifestations, we can hope to see such a reduction. But we have a long, long way to go.

# Appendix B: Sources of Additional Information

## Books

Lowinson, Joyce H., M.D., Pedro Ruiz, M.D., and Robert B. Millman, M.D., eds. *Substance Abuse: A Comprehensive Textbook*. 3rd. ed. Baltimore: Williams and Wilkins, 1997. (410-528-4000)

*American Psychiatric Association Practice Guidelines*. 1st ed. Washington, D.C.: American Psychiatric Association Press, 1996.
(202-682-6158)
Includes sections on the treatment of eating disorders and addiction to alcohol, cocaine, and opiates.

## Organizations

American Academy of Addiction Psychiatry
7301 Mission Rd.
Suite 252
Prairie Village, Kansas 66208
913-262-6161
fax: 913-262-4311
e-mail: addicpsych@aol.com
Web: www.aaap.org

American Society of Addiction Medicine
4601 North Park Avenue
Arcade Suite 101
Chevy Chase, Maryland 20815
301-656-3920
fax: 301-656-3815
e-mail: Email@asam.org
Web: www.asam.org

The Hazelden Foundation
PO Box 11
CO3
Center City, Minnesota 55012-0011
800-257-7810
The Hazelden Foundation has a bookstore and catalogue with many excellent references on all types of addiction.

Alcoholics Anonymous World Services, Inc.
Box 459
Grand Central Station, New York 10163
212-870-3400
Web: www.alcoholics-anonymous.org (note dash in Web address)
The AA central office has a catalogue of its official publications and pamphlets, including the Big Book of Alcoholics Anonymous.

National Council on Alcoholism and Drug Dependence, Inc.
12 West 21st Street
New York, New York 10010
212-206-6770
fax: 212-645-1690
e-mail: national@ncadd.org
Web: www.ncadd.org
Hope Line: 1-800-NCA-CALL (24 Hour Affiliate Referral)
The NCADD also has local offices in a hundred locations throughout the United States.

National Institute on Alcohol Abuse and Alcoholism (NIAA)
6000 Executive Boulevard
Willco Building
Bethesda, Maryland 20892-7003
Web: www.niaa.gov

NIAA Publications Distribution Center
attn: *Alcohol Alert*
PO Box 10686
Rockville, Maryland 20849-0686
*Alcohol Alert,* a free quarterly pamphlet prepared and distributed by the U.S. Department of Health and Human Services, is one of many resources available at NIAA.

National Institute on Drug Abuse (NIDA)
5600 Fishers Lane
Rockville, Maryland 20857
Web: www.nida.gov

NIDA Infofax
Science-based Facts on Drug Abuse and Addiction
1-888-NIH-NIDA (1-888-664-6432)
For the hearing impaired: 1-888-889-6432
NIDA also publishes a free research monograph series, as well as providing numerous sources of help and information.

Substance Abuse and Mental Health Services Administration (SAMHSA)
Center for Substance Abuse Treatment (CSAT)
5600 Fishers Lane
Rockville, Maryland 20857
Web: www.samhsa.gov
SAMHSA publishes a series of treatment improvement protocols (TIPS) that are available on request, as well as providing a wealth of additional information and resources.

*Pathological Gambling*

The National Council on Problem Gambling, Inc.
10025 Governor Warfield Pkwy.
Suite 311
Columbia, Maryland 21044

410-730-8008
fax: 410-730-0669
e-mail: ncpg@erols.com
Web: www.ncpgambling.com

Gamblers Anonymous International Service Office
PO Box 17173
Los Angeles, California 90017
213-386-8789
fax: 213-386-0030
e-mail: isomain@gamblersanonymous.org
Web: www.gamblersanonymous.org

*Eating Disorders*

American Anorexia Bulimia Association
165 West 46th Street
Suite 1108
New York, New York 10036
212 575 6200
Web: www.aabainc.org

Overeaters Anonymous World Services Office
6075 Zenith Court NE
Rio Rancho, New Mexico 87124
505-891-2664
fax: 505-891 4320
e-mail: overeatr@technet.nm.org

*Sexual Addiction*

Sex Addicts Anonymous
International Service Office of SAA
PO Box 70949
Houston, Texas 77270
1-800-477-8191
1-713-869-4902 (outside United States and Canada)

e-mail: info@saa-recovery.org
Web: sexaa.org

Incest Survivors Resource Network International
505-521-4260
e-mail: thehurtchild@zianet.com
Web: www.zianet.com/ISRNI

*For Families*

Al-Anon Family Group Headquarters, Inc.
1600 Corporate Landing Parkway
Virginia Beach, Virginia 23454
1-888-4AL-ANON (meeting information)
757-563-1600
fax: 753-563-1655
e-mail: wso@al-anon.org
Web: www.al-anon.alateen.org

National Alliance for the Mentally Ill
200 North Glebe Road
Suite 1015
Arlington, Virginia 22203-3754
1-800-950-NAMI (helpline)
703-524-7600
fax: 703-524-9094
TDD (Telecommunications Device for the Deaf): 703-516-7227
Web: www.NAMI.org

# Glossary

**Abstinence** A situation in which an addict avoids any use of drugs or alcohol and does not participate in addictive behaviors.

**Addictiveness** The measure of a substance's ability to produce changes in the brain that cause addiction.

**Analgesic** A drug used to relieve pain.

**Axon** A projection from a nerve cell that allows communication with another cell.

**Cell body** The main portion of a cell (for example, a nerve cell).

**Cell membrane** A complex sac surrounding a cell that is composed of various proteins and fats.

**Chronotropic** A drug effect that speeds up heart rate.

**Codependency** A coping strategy that involves abnormal investment in another person's problems; often seen in addicts' family members.

**Concordance** The degree to which genetically similar people, such as twins, share inherited characteristics.

**Conditioning** An unconscious learning process in which a stimulus gets paired with a physical response; important in drug cravings.

**Crack** A processed form of cocaine that is highly addictive.

**Delirium tremens** A state of altered consciousness and physical arousal that can occur during severe alcohol withdrawal.

**Delusions** Beliefs that are not based in reality (a person's culture must be taken into account on the question of whether or not a belief is delusional).

**Dementia** Loss of intellectual functioning.

**Denial** An unconscious defense mechanism in which an obvious reality is not believed; commonly seen in addiction.

**Designer drugs** Synthetically manufactured mood-altering drugs, often created to avoid legal regulation.

**Disinhibition** The loss of normal behavioral controls caused by the effects of mood-altering drugs.

**Dry drunk** A person who is abstaining from alcohol but who continues to be resentful and is not growing psychologically.

**Enabling** The (often unwitting) protection of an addict from the consequences of the addiction.

**Endorphin** A naturally produced substance found in the brain that resembles morphine and is involved in pain modulation and regulation of moods.

**Enzyme** A chemical whose purpose is to break down another chemical.

**Family history** A survey of diseases and disorders in the immediate or extended family of a patient, done to determine whether a person is at risk for an inherited disorder.

**Flashbacks** (1) The intrusive and involuntary reliving of a psychologically traumatic experience; (2) distortions in perception similar to those caused by hallucinogens that occur in former hallucinogen users from time to time long after use has stopped.

**Genetics** The study of the process of inheritance, including the structure of chromosomes and DNA.

**Half-life** The time it takes for half of the total amount of a drug to be broken down and eliminated from the system.

**Hallucinations** False perceptions in any sensory modality.

**Homeostasis** The tendency of a biological system to remain the same and to return to its previous state if disturbed.

**Intoxication** The effects on the body when a mood-altering drug is ingested.

**Intranasal** A way of taking a drug by sniffing it through the nose; the drug is absorbed through the tissue lining the inside of the nose.

**Intravenous** A way of taking a drug by injecting it into a blood vessel.

**Metabolism** The manner in which the body breaks down foods or drugs into smaller chemicals that are absorbed into the bloodstream and eliminated through the liver or kidney.

**Neurotransmitter** A specialized chemical that is secreted by a nerve cell for the purpose of attaching to a nearby nerve cell, thereby transmitting an electrical signal along the cell membrane.

**Paranoid** A term describing a person who believes that he or she is in danger when in reality no danger is present.

**Pharmacologic** Having to do with the chemical structure and metabolism of a drug.

**Physiological** Having to do with the function of body symptoms; physiological dependence is present when the body is physically dependent on a drug for normal functioning.

**Prognosis** The outlook for recovery from a disease or condition.

**Psychedelic** A term created in the 1960s to describe the experiences a person has when using hallucinogens such as LSD.

**Psychosis** A brain condition in which the person is out of touch with reality.

**Receptor** A component of a cell membrane that is designed to recognize and bind to a specific neurotransmitter.

**Reinforcement** A learning process (conscious or unconscious) that occurs when there is a pleasurable response to a given stimulus.

**Sedative** A drug that depresses brain functioning.

**Seizures** Unregulated electrical activity of brain cells.

**Skin conductance** The ability of the skin to modify a mild electrical charge; changes in proportion to how aroused or anxious a person is.

**Synapse** The gap between two nerve cells which contains neurotransmitters and receptors and is responsible for moving an electrical signal from cell to cell.

**Tolerance** A process in which the body develops an increased capacity to combat specific effects of a drug.

**Tranquilizer** A sedative drug that is designed to reduce anxiety levels; also known as an anxiolytic drug.

**White knuckling** The effort to avoid practicing an addiction simply by exerting will power.

**Withdrawal** A condition that occurs when an addictive drug is no longer present and the body systems come to be out of balance because of the adaptive changes that occurred when the body was developing tolerance (see **tolerance**).

# Index

Abstinence, 7
Abuse. *See* Psychological trauma
DSM-IV criteria, 4
in families of addicts, 86
substance, distinguished from dependence, 7–8, 9
Addiction
  costs to society, 170–71
  definition, 3–4
  development of, 16–21
  diagnosis, 4–8
  disorder of will, 11, 84, 91
  factors in development of
    agent, 18–19
    cultural, 8, 13
    environmental, 17–18
    host, 17
    moral model, 10
Addiction psychiatry, 111, 126, 139
Addiction Severity Index, 3
Addictive Personality, 32
Addictiveness
  definition, 18
  factor in development of addiction,
    9
Addictive disease
  concept, 10
  progression, 8
Adenosine, 48
Adrenaline, 29, 55. *See also* Norepinephrine; Sympathetic nervous
  system
Al-Anon. *See* Twelve-step programs
Al-Anon Family Group Headquarters,
  Inc., 192
Alcohol
  addictive properties of, 27, 48–49
  dementia, 51

depressant effects, 47
genetic differences in response to,
  49
induced coma, 48
intoxication, 47–48
respiratory arrest due to, 48
tolerance, 39–40
toxicity, 50–52
withdrawal, 41
Alcohol Alert, 190
Alcohol dehydrogenase, 26, 174–75
Alcohol dependence. *See* Alcoholism
Alcoholic cardiomyopathy, 51
Alcoholic hallucinosis, 51, 138
Alcoholics Anonymous, 7, 11, 114, 127–
  35. *See also* Twelve-step programs
  agnostics and atheists, 130–32
  anonymity, 132
  finding a meeting, 89, 135
  higher power, 130
  history, 127–28
  "spiritual awakening," 129
  spirituality, 128–32
  the Twelve Steps, 134
  useful sayings, 124–25
  Wilson, Bill, 127
"Alcoholics Anonymous" (the "Big
  Book"), 128, 129, 130, 131, 134, 182
Alcoholics Anonymous World Services,
  Inc., 189
Alcoholism
  continuous and episodic, 23
  definition, 4
  genetic research on, 175
  in pathological gambling, 155, 157
  medical consequences, 50–52
  type I and II, 23–24, 49